# The Cool Condom
## Compendium

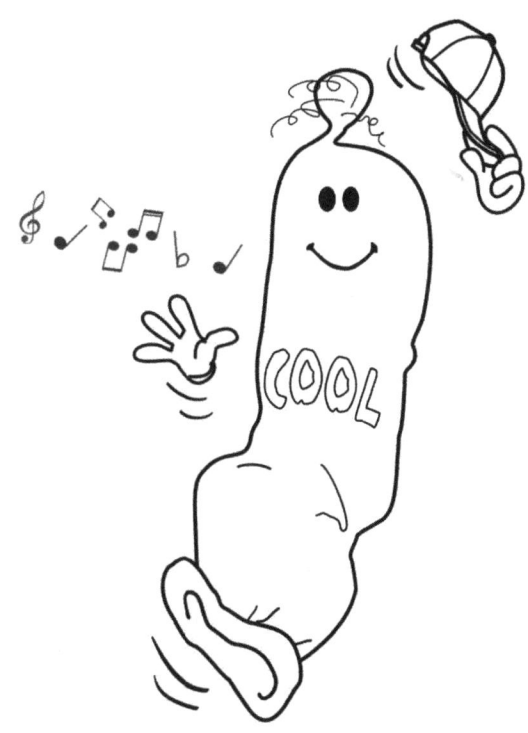

Johnnie Jazzemup

The Cool Condom Compendium
Copyright © 2018 Published by Jazzemup Creations

All rights reserved. No part of this book may be reproduced or transmitted in any form or by any means without written permission from the author.

ISBN-13: 978-0-9906975-5-8

Printed in USA by Create Space

# Contents

What Is A Condom ?.................. 8
A Brief History of the Condom....... 9 & 10
Condom Material Guide................ 11
So What Is Coming Next ?............ 12 & 13
Choosing the Correct Condom Size... 14 - 15
Instructions for a More Exacting Fit. 16
How to Put on a Condom.............. 17
Penis Particulars.................... 18 - 19
The Lowdown on Vaginas.............. 20 & 21
"G" Spot Q and A.................... 22 - 23
Condom Etiquette.................... 24
Anyone Up For Boppin Squiddles ?... 25
Lubes................................ 26
Spermicides......................... 27
Gazillions of Condom Idioms......... 28 - 29
Pubic Hair Facts.................... 30
Fashionable Pubic Hair.............. 31
Beware Vampire Pubic Crabs.......... 32
Prevention and Control.............. 33
Special Designer Condoms............ 34 & 35
Flavored Condoms.................... 36
Curious Condom Facts................ 37 - 39
Fun Condom Tips..................... 40 - 45
Foreign Words for Condoms........... 46
List of Elite Condom Patrons........ 47
Finger Length and Penis Size........ 48
Eye Watering Male Privates.......... 49
Fancy Names for Fancy Parts......... 50
Human Sperm Facts................... 51
Human Egg Facts..................... 52 - 53
Showers or Growers.................. 54
Erectile Disfunction/Impotence...... 55

Strange Forms of Ancient Birth Control. 56 - 57
Peyronie Problem.................... 58
Risky Sex........................... 59
Stiffy Lingo........................ 60
Wet Dreams and Flooding Nightmares. 61
Penis Park.......................... 62
Phallological Museum................ 63
What Makes a Good Lover ?........... 64
World's Best Lovers................. 65
Perfect Music for Quickies.......... 66 - 67
Slower Romantic Music Suggestions... 68 - 69
The 'OMG' Orgasm.................... 70 - 71
Blinded by The Night................ 72
Color a Condom...................... 73
Cool Condom Coloring Book........... 74
Sooty Sperm Discombobulations....... 75
Foreign Lingo for "Arriving"........ 76 - 77
15 Favorite Places to Make Out...... 78 - 79
Ups and Downs, Galloping the Maggot. 80
Stuffing the Envelope............... 81
Safe Sex is Good for You............ 82
Unsafe Sex is Not................... 83
STD/STI Statistics.................. 84
CDC Prevention Report 2017.......... 85
Chlamydia........................... 86
Syphilis............................ 87
Gonorrhea........................... 88
Gonorrhea Superbug.................. 89
HIV/AIDS............................ 90
HIV in the US....................... 91
HIV and Sex Education............... 92
Not Forgetting Our Environment...... 93
Warnings............................ 94

# Preface

Condoms have been around for a long, long time and they were probably in use thousands of years before the printing press came along and people learned to read instructions on their usage.

Communication on the subject was limited to the spoken word and I'm sure they were discussed at great length over a beer in old taverns by randy blokes who didn't have enough where-with-all to marry their partners raise families and consequently wanted to avoid having to confront those responsibilities at almost any cost.

Experimentation to avoid unwanted pregnancies must have been fierce as well as messy. Domestic life-stock with perfectly working intestines must have scattered in all directions when a party of young louts, eager to partake in the dirty deed, breezed confidently into town with sharpened knives at the ready.

Written instructions on the best made prophylactics and how best to conduct themselves in such matters of the "heart" were likely hanging on the walls of celibate monks in local monasteries as monks would have been the only ones around to read them even though they may well have been considered immoral. The local literate well-to-do may have sometimes scattered informative posters around towns and villages in the hope of preventing unwanted pregnancies and STDs but, the locals may have been more entertained by the crude pictures of curious looking phallic devices created from the many unsavory assorted materials that were graphically displayed on them.

Many books on contraception have been written since then of course but unwanted pregnancies as well as staggering rates of STDs still exist even though the general population can now read perfectly well and are, or should be, far more knowledgable about contraceptive use.

The idea of this book was conceived, if the word is appropriate, as a new "light hearted" approach that strives to prevent such unintentional occurrences, in a rather unconventional way. The Cool Condom Coloring book came first as just that, a coloring book. Every other topic for a coloring book seemed to have been explored already. Johnnie Jazzemup a world class doodler and time waster was eagerly looking for a completely unexplored new subject and he thought that adding a 3D element might add a new dimension to the world of coloring books. 3D tubular structures covered with random designs came to mind first and that initial concept very quickly evolved into the a whole new world of wacky condom fun, but still with serious undertones lurking quietly in the background.

It seemed to take forever but when the first book with such drawings was completed, the relevancy of a more informative book became more obvious. This cool and slightly irreverent book all about condoms seeks to fill that void. Condoms surround themselves with exquisite delights, humorous banter, wild and crazy facts and last but not least, some extremely serious reasons for regular use during sex.

# Introduction

As was stated in the preface, this compendium was created as a companion book to the Cool Condom Coloring Book. As you may well know, adult coloring books are exceedingly popular right now but the popularity of sex is catching up fast. Meticulously colored condoms are one thing but condoms and sex obviously affect every part of our lives and have a unique story all of their own so this condom companion book offers an opportunity to explore that side as well.

Various aspects of this intriguing story are told in this book with the help of the renowned writer of ludicrous and mostly unreadable books, Ivor Phewlines. Hence this playful book is replete with useful tips, fascinating facts, titllating tid bits, superfluous none-sense and wacky asides but besides the frivolity, it even includes a few extremely serious suggestions at the end just to cap off the party. The very humorous and artistic cartoons that accompany Ivor's stupefyingly inane scribblings were created by Connie Doms who skillfully integrated comical condoms into Ivor's meandering subject matter.

When you feel like a well earned break between reading this book and long periods of intense passion and lust, why not pick up a copy of the Cool Condom coloring book and get really creative with the old condom.

Relax and enjoy this wild and crazy compendium but, above all, whatever your sexual predilections are, be safe, and remember to use them whenever you indulge in the real thing. As Johnnie always says . . . "No balloons, no party."

Johnnie Jazzemup

Written by Ivor Phewlines<br>Cartoons by Connie Doms

# What is a Condom?

A condom is a thin piece of material that fits over a man's penis (male condom) or inside a woman's vagina (female condom) during sex. When used correctly, condoms prevent HIV, as well as pregnancy and sexually transmitted infections (STIs).

Sexual fluids such as semen, vaginal fluids and blood can transmit HIV and STIs. A condom forms a barrier between bodily fluids and entry points for HIV, such as: vagina, anus, penis (urethra), mouth.
Using a condom stops HIV: Use before any penetrative sexual activities, during vaginal, anal and oral sex, every time you have sex, on shared sex toys.

### There are Two Main Types of Condom.
The male condom is the most common type of condom. It fits around the penis.
The female condom is wider than the male condom, it fits inside the vagina or anus.

### Male Condoms come in Various Shapes and Sizes

Standard condoms have straight sides. Fitted condoms are indented below the head of the penis.
Large condoms are longer and wider giving more room. Some condoms are wider over the head of the penis. Extra strong condoms are thicker - important for anal sex. Textured condoms, with ribs or bumps, can increase sensation for both partners. Colored or flavored condoms can make oral sex more yummy.

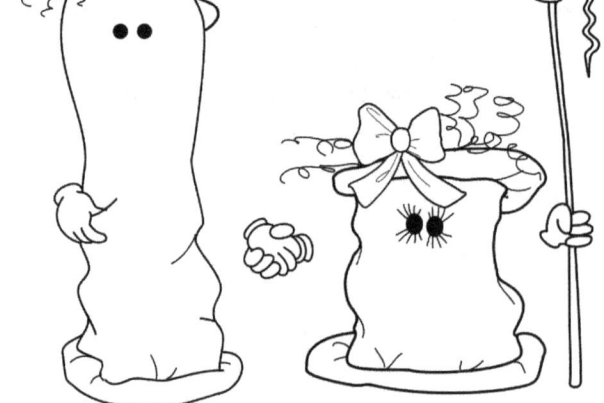

### If the Condom Breaks During Sex...
Withdraw the penis immediately and use a new condom.
Access emergency contraception if not using other contraceptive methods.
Both partners should be tested for HIV and STIs.
Access emergency HIV treatment if you are at risk of HIV infection.

### Condom Effectiveness
Condoms are very effective at protecting against HIV, other STIs and pregnancy.
Use a new condom every time you have sex.
Always use extra water-based lubricant during anal sex.
Use certified condoms E.g. FDA, CE, ISO, Kitemark.

**Some STIs are transmitted by skin-to-skin contact so condoms cannot protect you from these.**

# A Brief History of the Condom

Of course we all know that sex was originally invented in a secluded orchard situated in a garden called Eden that contained a forbidden tree. The orchard was inhabited by a crafty serpent who initiated the exchange of a rotten apple between two nudists, one of whom had previously popped out of the dust and the other that subsequently sprang from one of his ribs. But the question here is, when were condoms invented ?

Apparently a good while after the aforementioned event, around 11,000-13,000 years ago there are signs that condoms were in use. The first evidence of condoms appeared in France with a painting on the wall of a cave that supposedly represents the very very first one.

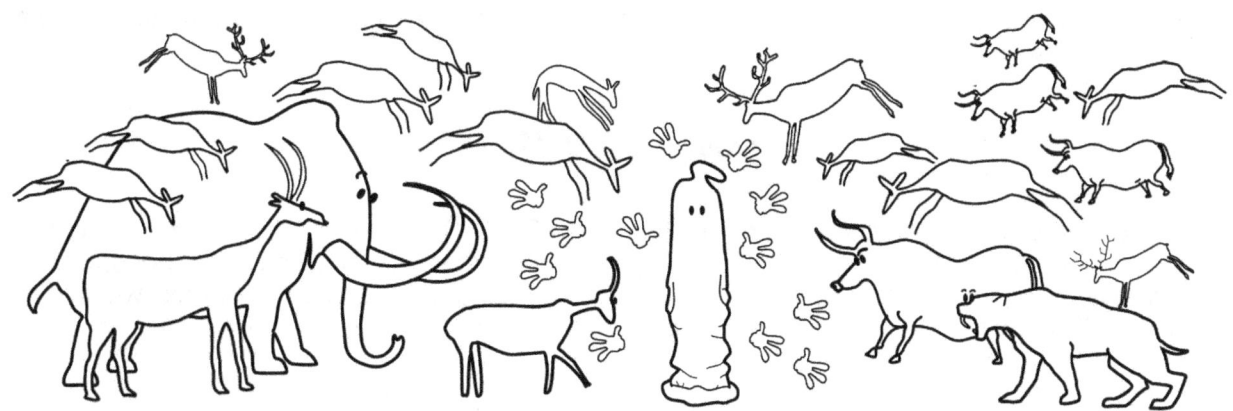

In ancient Egypt at around 1000 B.C. condoms made from cloth were used to protect against disease.

Glans condoms, that only covered the head of the penis, were invented in China and Japan during the 1400s A.D. The Chinese used lamb intestines or oiled silk paper and in Japan they used tortoise shells or animal horns.

In the 1500s Gabrielle Fallopius and Italian physician wrote about the frequently fatal STD syphilis. He recommended the use of a protective linen sheath, soaked in chemicals and dried in order to prevent catching this disease.

In 1605 a Catholic theologian declared that condoms were immoral.

Moving along to the 1600s condoms were made from animal intestines and made available to the public if they could afford them. However in 1666 when the birth rate dropped the English Birth Rate Commission blamed it on "condons" the first time the word was published.

Later on in 1700s condoms became more reliable. They were made of either intestine or bladder treated with sulfur or lye or linen soaked in chemicals, and were sold in public places, like pubs, markets or from crudely created condom vending machines.

In early 1800s people publicly began advocating condoms for birth control and in 1839 Charles Goodyear created rubber condoms which led to the word "rubber" for a "condom." There are now many words for condoms and they are listed on pages 28 and 29.

In 1918 a judge "somewhere" ruled that condoms could be advertised and sold to prevent STDs.

The sales of condoms nearly doubled during the 1920s and in 1927-31 they were made standard issue for the military.

"No ballons ? No party !" came along for the 42% of Americans who relied on them for birth control and prevention of STDs.

In 1957 Durex introduced the first lubricated condom.

When the AIDs epidemic started in the 1980s condom use rose substantially and now in 2017 we can now purchase condoms in a variety of shapes, flavors, textures, colors and materials.

## Moldy Oldies

The world's oldest surviving condom dates back to 1640 and is on display in an Austrian museum. This Swedish condom is made of pig intestine and was said to be soaked in warm milk prior to use to ensure it was disease free. Other ancient condoms were made of oiled silk paper, animal bladders, tortoise shells, fish skin, and animal horns.

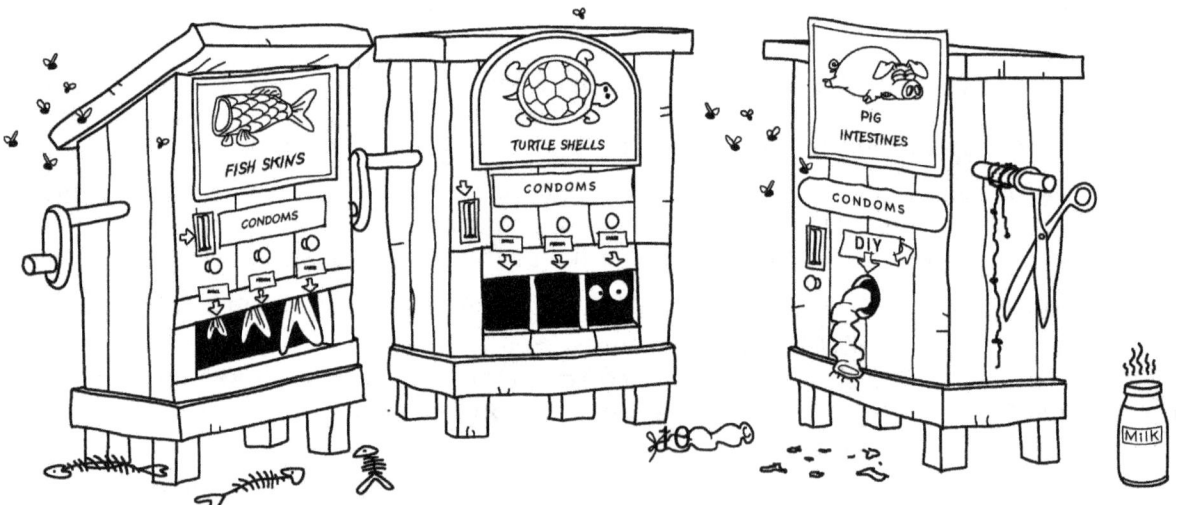

Primitive designs for early condom vending machines.

# Condom Material Guide

Condom materials have come a long way since the early days of the very first cloths, animal intestines and the later Goodyear condoms. Today Latex condoms can stretch up to 800% it's size although I'm not at all sure why as there must be few humans who need them that size? There is of course a latex allergic response problem that exists for some people so obviously they should steer well clear of latex and use condoms made from other materials instead. These materials are :-

## Polyurethane

A polyurethane condom is probably the most popular alternative to latex. Polyurethane is of a type of plastic that conducts heat better than latex and it is also thinner, which many men find to be more pleasurable. Some female condoms are also made of polyurethane.

## Polyisoprene

This product is another alternative for those who have a latex allergy. It contains many of the same properties as latex but not the same materials that can cause an allergic reaction. They tend to be a little cheaper than polyurethane but they are a little thicker. Most people can't even notice because polyisoprene condoms are softer, stretchier, and feel more natural than rubber.

## Lambskin

Up until recently, lambskin condoms have been the only alternative for those with a latex allergy. They are not actually made of lambskin, but a layer of membrane from inside of a sheep's intestines called the cecum. People have been using animal gut like cecum to make condoms for hundreds of years because it's very durable, thin, and they conduct heat really well. However lambskin condoms DO NOT protect against viral STDs/STIs like herpes or HIV.

## Nitrile

The latest generation of female condoms are made of a type of rubber called nitrile. Nitrile is also used for disposable rubber gloves for those with a latex allergy, so they are a great option for those who have one. Because they're made of nitrile, female condoms are oil-resistant, meaning that they can handle oil-based lube like vaseline or baby oil without breaking down.

# So...What is Coming Next?

With many still the design stage there are brand new technological developments in the works with quite a few new condom prototype designs that will improve safety and make sex with a mores sensitive condom even more pleasurable.

## The Galactic Cap
Sits on the head of the penis rather than covering the shaft. It is described as easier to apply, safer and more secure, while allowing for more pleasure.

## The Graphene Condom
Graphene is a type of carbon that is a single atom thick. Condoms made from this material must be about as thin as they will ever get without having to pay good money for a "nothing there at all" condom !

## Project Rapidom
A condom with applicator handles which enables a man to put it on quickly and correctly especially in low light.

## Ultra-Sensitive Reconstituted Collagen Condom
A condom created to feel like a second skin, a reinvention of a leather condom using using collagen fibers from bovine tendons.

## The I-Con Smart Condom
The i.Con Smart Condom is being billed as the newest form of wearable technology. It is worn at the base of a real condom and is adjustable for size. It can be worn multiple times. and using nano-chip and Bluetooth technology it relays data to a smart phone app.

According to British Condoms this ring is lightweight and water resistant. The inbuilt technology provides a range of capabilities for providing a range of statistics on a person's most intimate moments in order to improve their sex lives.

This includes duration, speed, and girth measurements as well as the amount of calories burned and different positions. It can even detect chlamydia and syphilis.

i.Con Smart Condom will measure:

Calories burned during sexual intercourse
Speed of thrusts
Total number of thrusts
Frequency of sessions
Total duration of sessions
Average velocity of thrusts
Girth measurement
Average skin temperature

Different positions used (currently BETA testing.
I-Con will have more info in a release coming soon.)

The ring has an integrated micro USB port so it can be recharged, with each charge lasting about six to eight hours. It also comes with a one year warranty.

British Condoms has been delivering condoms and other products since 1999. Last year it revealed that it was developing the unique product.

Adam Leverson, lead engineer on the i.Con project said: 'Not only have we innovated the world's first smart condom ring - that'll measure pretty much every aspect of performance in the bedroom - but now I'm pleased to confirm that it will also have built-in indicators to alert the users to any potential STIs present.'

The firm claims 90,000 people have already pre-ordered the product which will be released later this year at the price of £59.99 ($80.99).

## The Silicone Condom

Condoms are usually made of latex, but silicone condoms offer a loose fit that is pulled on as you would a mitten instead of being rolled on. The condoms are lubricated on the inside in order to provide men with a more pleasurable sensation.

Because silicone is thicker and stronger than latex, it holds a better form than latex or any other current condom material. Just because it's thicker doesn't mean it will reduce sensation. These condoms are designed to be provide stimulation from the inside instead of from the outside in, pleasing both parties.

## Origami Condoms

Origami condoms which are the first non-rolled, injection- molded, engineered, silicone condom, are supposedly due to be released at some point in the future.

The controversy over the potential release date of this much anticipated condom continues as legal battles between Origami condom inventor Daniel Resnic, his former employee, and the National Institute of Health (NIH) rages on.

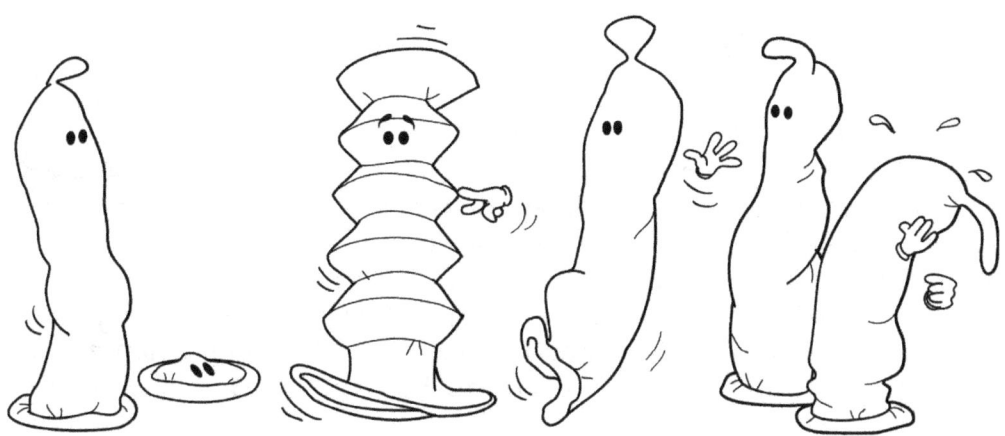

# Choosing the Correct Condom Size

## Simplest Method

Choosing the right condom is simple really. The best tip is to take the cardboard tube off an empty toilet paper roll and slide it over a full hard-on. If there's extra room, your best bet is a smaller condom. Just enough room means you're at a medium, and if the cardboard tube is too tight for you, opt for a large.

Fiddling around with a ruler in a drug store while you are trying to figure out what size condom size you need to purchase is a definite no, no.

## Other Method

To calculated the condoms Circumference (girth) the flat width of the condom is doubled. Example a condom with a 2.3" width would have a circumference of 4.6" If you are looking for a wider condom, pay attention to the width measurement on a condom size chart many of which are available online. Instructions for a more exact fit are on page 16.

## Exaggerations !

A survey by dating website SaucyDates.com reveals the countries where men exaggerate the most about the size of their penis - and those where they are too modest.

The results show that Australian men are the worst offenders when it comes to exaggeration.

American men are also prone to overselling their wares. Brits were almost as bad.

Canadians were the most honest and men in India actually underestimated the size of their manhood.

## Tight Fit !!!

Roberto Esquivel Cabrera, 54, from Saltillo, Mexico, has a penis measuring a colossal 18.9 inches when flaccid which touches his knee. Roberto made headlines worldwide in 2015 after a video went viral showing him weighing his member to prove its authenticity.

His half-meter penis smashed the unofficial record believed to belong to US actor Jonah Falcon, whose penis was 9.5 inches flaccid and 13.5 inches when erect.

The Guinness Book of Records doesn't recognize this kind of record however.

## Does Size Count ?

When it comes to penises, size does matter — at least for some women. Women who are more likely to have vaginal orgasms say it is easier to orgasm with men who have longer penises, according to a 2012 study published in the Journal of Sexual Medicine.

In a 2013 study detailed in the journal Proceedings of the National Academy of Sciences, researchers reported women said the ideal penis size varied with a man's height, with a larger organ looking better on taller men.

According to studies for one-night stands, size does matter, but it's not penis length that women are concerned about, apparently it's the girth that matters!

## Smaller Condoms ?

News just in....The FDA backs move to make smaller 'bespoke' condoms because the average size of 6.69 inches is TOO BIG for American men so they keep slipping off.

The average erect penis size in America is 5.57 inches, about an inch shorter than the standard condom size.

Experts think that this might be one of the main reasons why just one-third of single American men use a condom during sex.

The Food and Drug Administration, which regulates health industry standards, has conceded that there is a need for smaller condoms in a desperate bid to lower the rates of sexually transmitted diseases and unwanted pregnancies.

The standard condom is between 6.7 and 8.3 inches long, and around 4.1 inches in width.
Data collated by "ONE" Condoms found condoms only fit 12 percent of men. The rest have varying widths and lengths that are not covered by the one-size-fits-all approach.

This corresponds with the latest scientific research. The most high-profile study, conducted by Dr Debby Herbenick at Indiana University, asked 1,661 men in the U.S. to give the size of their penis. The study documented varying lengths - from 1.5 inches to just over 10 inches.

The research team found that the size of the erect penis varied depending on how it was achieved. Oral sex proved more arousing than masturbation or being stimulated only by sexual fantasies.

"ONE" Condoms offers 60 different dimensions, from 4.9 to 9.4 inches in length and from 3.5 to 5.0 inches in width. Whatever your size "ONE" Condoms has a bespoke condom for you that will fit perfectly.

# Instructions for a More Exacting Fit

Length is important to make sure the condom covers the whole of your shaft. If the condom is too long, it's going to bunch up at the base, which looks odd and can act like a tourniquet (rubber band) causing tightness. On the other hand, if the condom is too short then it's not going to cover you fully, and may be pulled off during sex. That's clearly not a good thing either. So "TheyFit" offers 12 different condom lengths, starting at 80mm (3") and rising to 240mm (9.5").

Circumference is important to make sure your condom stays securely in place during sex, while still being comfortable. A circumference that is too small is going to feel tight, and uncomfortable. You may lose your erection, or have difficulty reaching orgasm (most guys report not being "able to feel anything" during sex - this is caused by the tightness). On the other hand, a circumference that's too big will be loose and could slip, or fall off entirely. That's bad too. TheyFit" offer 14 different condom circumferences, suitable for girths from 3.2", up to 7.5", factoring in the perfect amount of stretch for each fitting.

Multiple scientific studies dating as far back as 1993 have all identified that between 40-45% of men have problems finding a condom that fits. Problems like the condom slipping, or falling off. Problems like a condom feeling tight, or uncomfortable, or stopping you being able to orgasm.

Length is important to make sure the condom covers the whole of your shaft. If the condom is too long, it's going to bunch up at the base, which looks odd and can act like a tourniquet (rubber band) causing tightness. On the other hand, if the condom is too short then it's not going to cover you fully, and may be pulled off during sex. That's clearly not a good thing either. "TheyFit" offers 12 different condom lengths, starting at 80mm (3") and rising to 240mm (9.5").

The circumference measurement is important to make sure your condom stays securely in place during sex, while still being comfortable. A circumference that is too small is going to feel tight, and uncomfortable. You may lose your erection, or have difficulty reaching orgasm (most guys report not being "able to feel anything" during sex - this is caused by the tightness). On the other hand, a circumference that's too big will be loose and could slip, or fall off entirely which is not a good idea.

"TheyFit" offer 14 different condom circumferences, suitable for girths from 3.2", up to 7.5", factoring in the perfect amount of stretch for each fitting.

# How To Put On A Condom

Try practicing with a banana first if you need to but remember to be gentle with it!

**1.** Always check the expiration date on the wrapper.

**2.** Carefully tear the packet using the serrated edge, but be careful of sharp nails, jewelry, scissors or your teeth.

**3.** You need to make sure that the condom is the right way up because condoms can only roll on in one direction effortlessly. The reservoir needs to face away from the tip of the penis before you put it on. Squirting just a little water based lubricant inside the tip can enhance your sensation even more but don't overdo it. Squeeze the reservoir end so that no air is trapped inside (the condom may split otherwise) and place it over the head of a completely hard weenie. Make sure the condom fits snugly over this weenie.

**4.** If you are uncircumcised, pull back the foreskin before keeping one hand at the head of the penis with the teat of the condom between your forefinger and thumb, and use the other to roll the condom on all the way down the shaft to the base. If you have problems with a condom that will not unroll, it is probably on inside out so start again with a new condom, as there may be sperm on it.

**5.** This is a good point to rub some water-based lubricant to the outside of the condom. This is an especially good idea if you are not using a pre-lubricated one, and even if you are, using extra lubricant increases sensitivity and helps to avoid any breakages.

**6.** If the condom rolls back up during sex you just need to roll it back down. If it comes off, you need to put on a new one. After you have finished be sure to hold the condom at the base of your weenie while you are still erect before you pullout to make sure it doesn't slip off.

Take the condom off when your penis is completely withdrawn.

**7.** After use, tie a knot in the condom so that none of the contents spill out. Carefully wrap it in a tissue and put it in a waste bin.

**Never flush it down a toilet!**

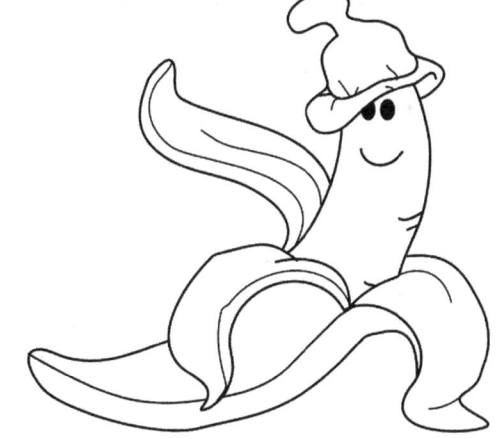

# Penis Particulars

## Where Did The Name Penis Come From ?
The word "penis" is taken from the Latin word for "tail." Prior to that it was called a "yard".

## Night Time Erections
Healthy men typically experience between three and five erections during a night's sleep with each one typically lasting for 25-30 minutes. That's like four hours of nightly erections. Whew....

## Unaligned Round Objects
One testicle always hangs a little lower than the other so they don't bounce off each other and make a curious knocking sounds when a dude is walking down the street.

## Oversize Feet
Large feet do not correspond to large packages so, when a single girl is finished checking out a prospective suitors watch, it is not necessary to check out the size of his feet as well. Just kidding :)

## Recovery
After an orgasm, a man might still be up but he usually needs around 20 minutes time out. Some may even need all day to recover, some even longer than that.

## Early Starters
Did you know that baby boys can get erections in the womb - ultrasounds have proved it. Maybe the bumps a pregnant woman experiences are not just caused by elbows and knees.

## Flexible
The penis is not a muscle, there are none there at all so forget it guys, working it out in a gym wan't improve the looks of it. Apparently the darn thing can bend as much as a boomerang although Australia is not the only place where this feat is performed.

## Strong Sperm
Spanish researchers showed pictures of men who had good, average and not so good sperm to a group of women..They were then instructed to pick out the best looking men and, guess what ? These women most often chose the ones who produced the best sperm.

## Brainless Wonder
The order to ejaculate comes from the spinal cord. No brain is necessary for ejaculation.

## Size
For those that still worry about such trivialities, here's another reassuring thing, vaginas typically adjust themselves to any size or length.Women are around 85% totally satisfied with their partner's contribution.For eye watering male privates in the Animal Kingdom check out page 49.

## Short Changed
The average male orgasm lasts 6 seconds. Women get 23 seconds. What a swizz !

## Circumcision
30% of men over the age of 15 have been circumcised which was started by the 19th century middle classes on either side of the Atlantic who were hysterical about masturbation and thought circumcision would cure it.

## Short On The Calories
Semen contains only one to seven calories which is less than a half cup of summer squash at 10 calories.

## Starting Out The Same
Who would have thought that once upon a time penises and clitorises started out the same? During the first eight weeks from conception in the womb, the undifferentiated genital group of cells start forming into either one or the other depending on the embryo receiving 'male' hormones, or not.

## Painful Uncoupling
A man's penis is not a real bone and can actually break, swell and go all blue when it does. If it is twisted hard enough or subjected to too much uncontrolled action while on top, the blood vessels that supply the scaffolding for the erection can burst. A third of these accidents are caused by a sudden and unexpected uncoupling so take care and don't let your passion get completely out of control !

## The Short And The Long Of It
According to German researchers, the average intercourse session lasts 2 minutes, 50 seconds. Oddly women perceive it as lasting 5 minutes, 30 seconds ?????

## Well Worn Dicks.
A phallus is a penis, especially when erect or an object that resembles a penis, or a make believe image of an erect penis. They have been represented just like todays graffiti for eons by many civilizations in all parts of the world.

A 28,000-year-old siltstone phallus discovered in the Hohle Fels cave is among the oldest phallic representations known but there are many others examples scattered throughout the globe in artwork, statues, carvings and petroglyphs created by many diverse people.

In Brazil's Lapa do Santo Rock Shelter, a huge artistic manifestation of a phallus in the form of a petroglyph was discovered pecked onto rocks and dated to be between 9,000 and 12,000 years old.

On the limestone cliffs of a remote Greek island, Astypalaia in the Aegean, dick inscriptions were discovered that not only represented inscribed penises but also expressed in large letters sexual desire and even the act itself. The carvings date from the fifth and sixth centuries B.C. These ancient Greeks used to record just who was having sex with whom.

## The Fear Factor
Phallophobia is the fear of a penis. I'm not sure how a person handles that.

# The Lowdown on Vaginas

## Where Does The Name Vagina Come From ?
"Vagina" comes from the Latin root meaning "sheath for a sword." So there, now you know !

## The Vagina Is A Self-Cleaning Organ
Great for those ladies that have already had enough just cleaning the house, the vagina produces its own protective substances to get rid of unwanted fluids and bacteria. It's best to let it clean itself naturally than use feminine hygiene products that can put your natural pH out of balance.

## Women Can Also Ejaculate
It is rare occurrence and the exact mechanics of how it all works are not fully understood. A liquid comprised of glucose, prostatic acid phosphatise as well as two ingredients found in urine supposedly build up in the spongy tissue of the G-Spot. When it is repeatedly stimulated it can come shooting out of the urethra.

## Having Babies Doesn't Make A Vagina Noticeably Different
Apparently, according to statistical research done in 1996, having a baby does not alter vaginal size.

## The Clitoris Resembles A Wishbone
Research has shown that the clitoris has branches that extend down underneath the skin on the sides of the vulva in a wishbone shape. It is also 80% the size of a penis and wraps around the back of the vagina.

## Roughly Half Of American Women Use Vibrators
Americans spend $15 billion on sex toys annually, that 44 percent of women 18 to 60 have used one. 78 percent of those women were in a relationship when they did. Over a third said they used one during intercourse and 41% during foreplay.

## A Dedicated Follower Of Passion
A clitoris has one function only and that is to provide pleasure and how ! It has an estimated 8,000 nerve endings which is the densest nerve supply of any organ in the the female body. Males have nothing that compares with it. Sadly refunds are not available to guys who feel they have been short changed.

## Vage Museum
A feminist YouTuber Florence Schechter is crowdfunding to bring the world's first Vagina Museum to London. This fascinating museum will be a showcase for Science, Culture, Society and History. It will also offer Community Outreach, Policy Work, Numerous Exciting Events, Gallery and even a cafe. There is no physical vagina building yet but this new Muffs Museum is apparently 'stirring" and getting all warmed up ready to go.

## A Little Bit Of A Tilt
A vagina is tilted at around a 130-degree angle but this can flatten out a bit with age and menopause.

## Sizes Shapes And Colors
There is no such thing as a standard vulva or vagina, they come in all sorts of different shapes and colors. There are even art galleries that display full color enlarged photos of every description for the public to view.

## More Orgasms
Lesbians report that they have more orgasms than straight or bisexual women according to the Journal of Sexual Medicine that surveyed 6,151 men and women.

## Live Yogurt And Thrush
A fungal infection called thrush in the vagina is pretty common in women but why they get it isn't exactly unclear. It is usually uncomplicated and about 75% of women get it in their lifetime usually occurring in a woman's reproductive years.
Usually it was recommended that a dab of live yogurt in their vagina would clear it up. Alas it has been discovered that the lactobacilli in yogurt is not the kind that is best for your vagina. So maybe forget the yogurt, anti-fungal medication is really the best solution is symptoms persist.

## Size Doesn't Matter
The average vagina is only around 3 to 4 ins size but when aroused it can stretch to twice that length.

## Take It To The Gym
In 2009, Tatyana Kozhevnikova reportedly set the vagina weightlifting record by lifting 31 pounds. She attached the weight to a wooden egg so her muscles could grab onto it. No mention of a spotter and no mention in the Guinness Book of Records either.

## An Orgasm Can Be More Affective Than A Painkiller
When you have an orgasm your body releases a stream of brain chemicals called endorphins which are a kind of natural morphine, feelings of euphoria follow.

## Caught In The Act
Ever heard of penis captivus ? This happens when muscles in the vagina clamp down so hard on a penis it makes it impossible to withdraw. Yikes, thank goodness it is very rare. I can't imagine how embarrassing it must be to call 911 to report the problem. A few dozen police cars, an ambulance and a street fill of neighbors might be too much to deal with.

## No Orgasms ?
According to one study around 16% of women say they have never had an orgasm during intercourse and 20-30% say they only reached orgasm during sex about one in four times.

# "G" Spot Q and A

## What is the G spot ?

The **G-spot** is also called the Gräfenberg **spot** after the German gynecologist Ernst Gräfenberg who discovered it in the 1940s and actually described it as a a zone. It is characterized as an erogenous area of the vagina that, when stimulated, may lead to strong sexual arousal, powerful orgasms and potential female ejaculation.

This spot is elusive because many scientists are not even sure it exists. There is a lot of anecdotal evidence and reliable reports that say this specific area does exist but not much in the way of anatomical proof. Some women love this amazing magic button and others are mystified by it.

## Where is it ?

Apparently this controversial and fabled pleasure location is roughly about 2 inches inside the frontal, anterior, belly button side of the vagina but will obviously vary depending on the physical attributes of each woman and the type of topographical map consulted. The distance between a belly button and the top of a pelvic bone can differ quite a bit between different women.

## What does the actual "G-spot" feel like ?

If you feel a ribbed or texture area you are close, if you feel a bean shaped bump you are spot on. The spot is composed of tissue that swells when it becomes aroused and is easier to find when a woman is turned on.

## Can I use other letters of the alphabet besides just plain old G ?

While the G-spot may not even exist there are new spots that might, at least according to Italian researchers.They say there is a highly secret place that researchers call the "clitourethrovaginal" complex, maybe a C+2 spot, which is a serious pleasure point that creates even longer lasting experiences that radiate throughout the entire body. This actually describes the area that includes the clitoris, vagina and urethra. With two contenders vying for the top erogenous zones, the G -spot and the clitoris. Is this new third contender meeting spot going to make everything even more complicated ? Well, sexologists and other researchers disagree with the study's findings and thinks it lacks validity.

But now, just to make things even more complicated an "A-Spot has been discovered and is called The Anterior Fornix Erogenous Zone located in a tender bit of tissue at the end of your vagina and just in front of the cervix.Maybe it's all getting getting a bit overwhelming. Maybe not thinking about it too much and just getting on with it might be the best way to deal with all these elusive spots.

## What are the two types of orgasm for women?

Well, a man is aroused quickly has a brief orgasm and immediately falls into the refractory phase which is usually sleep sometimes even losing some interest in his partner along the way. A bucket of cold water by the bed might be the best solution ladies.

A woman, on the other hand, can experience two types of orgasm, a clitoral and vaginal. A clitoral is similar to a man's which is short, sharp peak which loses energy and arousal quickly. The clitoris can also become hyper sensitive and unbearable to touch.

The second way, a vaginal orgasm retains energy and can spread pleasure throughout the entire body. This version is usually caused by stimulation of the G or other elusive spots. Feelings of euphoria, joy and relief are often used to describe the experience G Spot climax. Supposedly it is more intense and more complete with more depth and meaning.

## How do these spots and zones help when they are all revved up?

Supposedly, when located, activated and expertly manipulated, they all facilitate a blissful orgasm that drives a woman wild and crazy with exulted orgasmic exultations that can even spread to the upper areas of the body and sometimes the entire universe as well.

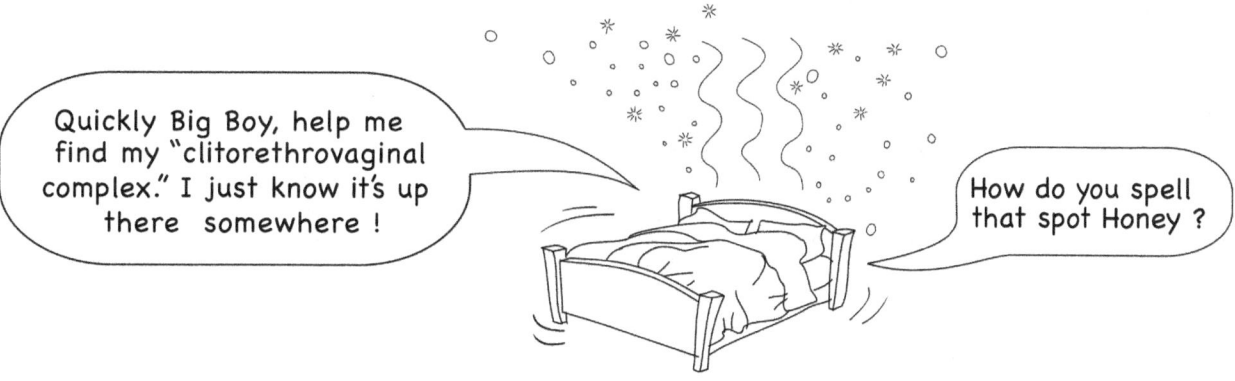

Of course there is is no reason to stop exploring and discovering new spots of the alphabet if you desire. Why not try out a few more letters if you like just to see what happens. Do your own personal research, keep detailed notes, time charts, graphs, sketches and map drawings next to the bed and maybe you too can start new rumors about new unexplored alphabetical letters that really do work deliciously at newly discovered spots in your own private landscape of female sexual wonderment, awe and ecstasy.

# Condom Etiquette

**Etiquette is the customary code of polite behavior in society or in bed.**

While condoms are available in a wide variety of styles and textures, it is considered thoughtless and immature to introduce extreme variations like "the dinosaur design" first time out, especially with an inexperienced partner.

- Regardless of how casual a sexual encounter may be, it is considered tactless and crude to dispose of the condom in a manner which could only construed as thoughtless, lazy or a newly contrived olympic event.
- When it has been determined that a sexual encounter will NOT take place, it is rude to employ the condom as a device for amusement., like drawing a face on it and using it as a finger puppet for instance.
- Most condoms are packaged with a complete set of instructions but it is considered rude and improper to read them immediately prior to use especially if you are a slow reader and like to mouth the words as you are reading.
- While it is not inappropriate for one's partner to apply the condom, it is simply a matter of courtesy to insure that sufficient lighting is provided to prevent stumbling around in the dark and possibly having it end up on the cat's tail.
- It is appropriate to offer one's partner a choice of colors when selecting condoms but special care should be taken to insure that this option is not presented in an untimely fashion such as the moment you pick them up at their front door on your very first date.
- Care should always be taken to insure that used condom wrappers are properly disposed of. A trash can full of used condom wrappers or even a pile of used condoms hanging off your bed table is not the best way to impress a new partner.
- It is considered rude, untimely and a definite passion damper to make one's partner wait for a few hours while figuring out the intricacies of using a new condom.

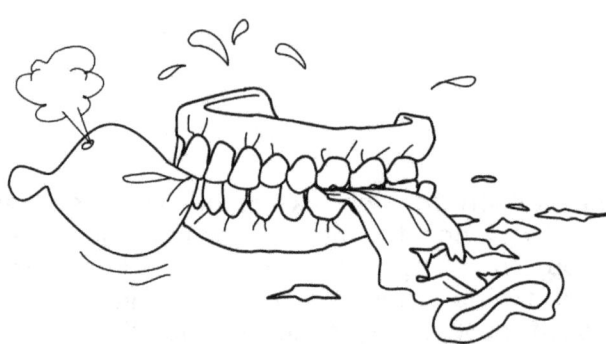

- Do not open a condom wrapper with one's teeth in order to avoid the accidental destruction of its contents or the unanticipated ejection of your dentures.

# "Anyone Up For Boppin' Squiddles?"

Organ Grinding
Skinning the Cat
Moving Furniture
Rolling in the Hay
Winding the Clock
Furgling
The Lust and Thrust
Hiding the Bishop
How's your Father
Plowing Through the Bean Field
Doing the Dirty Deed
Nookie
Getting One's Banana Peeled
Grummeting
Baking the Potato
Hanky Panky
Giving the Dog a Bone
Having it Off
Buttering the Biscuit
Introducing Charlie
Jumping the Turnstile
The Hokey-Pokey
Getting One's Kettle Mended
Fidgeting the Midget in Bridget
Crashing the Custard Truck
Doodling
Having Pot Pudding for Dinner
Shrimping the Barbie
Paddling up Coochie Creek
Tubular Wedging
Threading the Needle
Doing the Horizontal Greased-Weasel Tango
Extreme Flirting
Kalamanga
Playing a Game of Mr. Wobbly
Bump and Grind
Playing with the Box the Kids Came in
Burying the Burrito
Roasting the Broomstick
Feeding the Kitty
Searching for Pocket Change
Boppin' Squiddles
Putting the Banana in the Fruit Salad
Whitewashing the Picket Fence
Bringing an Al Dente Noodle to the Spaghetti House
Banging
Weinering
Taking the Bald-Headed Gnome for a Stroll in the Misty Forest
Daubing the Brush
Basket Weaving
Shagging
Rumpty Pumpy
Canoodling
Frigging
Bonking

Digging up the Sand Crab

# Lubes

Lubes are not just for older women who have lost their natural lubrication later in life. Apparently 30% of women suffer from natural dryness even when aroused at any age. This varies due to hormonal levels which change with their cycles. Lube reduces the risk of tearing and injury if rough or anal sex is on your agenda. There are many textures, flavors and sensations to try which will only add more fun to your tasty sexual menu. Just remember to play Simon and Garfunkle's "Slip Sliding Away" as background music while trying out your lube experiments.

Although condoms are usually lubricated with long lasting sex they can dry out and a dry condom is a condom that can more easily break. The anus doesn't naturally lubricate so it is even more important to lubricate when taking that route to pleasure. Starting out with a few drops is recommended and adding more if needed is a good idea. This is all down to what you are doing, using a condom or not, foreplay, massages and whatever you are dong sexually. Always use it with sex toys although be careful not to use silicone lubricants with a toy that is silicone-based because they can be damaged. Use a water based lube instead. Basically oil based lubes are not compatible with condoms because it makes the porous and obviously less safe to use.

You may even be allergic to your lube so test it out on a small patch of your skin before using it.

Oil-based lubricants can change the pH balance in the vagina, possibly increasing your risk of infection. Previous research has found that mineral oils can reduce a latex condom's strength by approximately 90 percent.

**Just remember that lube is NOT a spermicide and will not prevent STDs or pregnancies either.**

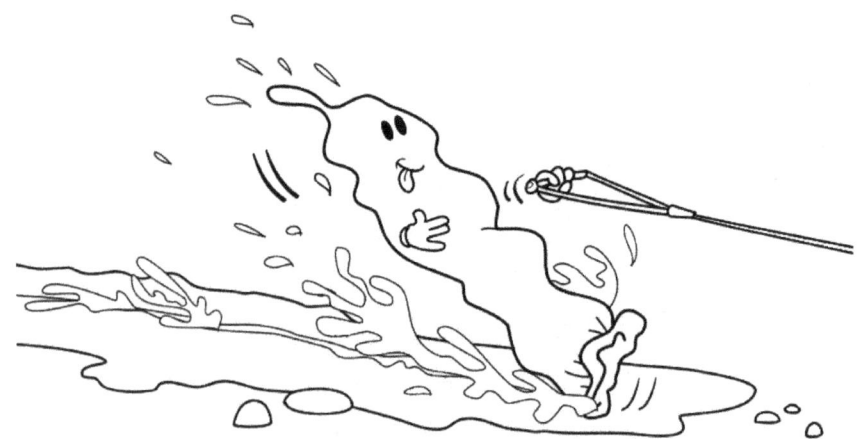

# Spermicides

Spermicide is a contraceptive substance that immobilizes and destroys sperm before they can swim into the uterus. It is inserted vaginally prior to intercourse to prevent pregnancy. The most common spermicides are available in many forms, such as jelly (gel), films, and foams. Be sure to read the instructions on the packaging and check the expiration date. Spermicide is affordable, convenient, easy to use, and hormone-free.

### Boost
It can be used alone but is more effective with other birth control methods.

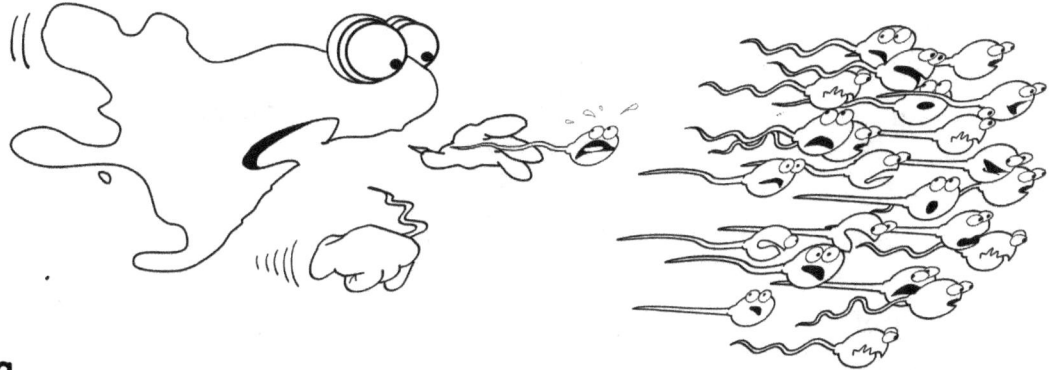

### Timing
Timing is important when it comes to spermicide. Some spermicide isn't effective right away and must inserted with your fingers like a tampon at least 10-15 minutes before sex. And many spermicides are only effective for 1 hour after you put them in your vagina. If you're going to have sex more than once, you'll need to add more spermicide. But using spermicide several times a day can cause irritation that increases your risk for STDs, so it's a good idea to use condoms to protect yourself.

### Pros
Easy to use and convenient to get a hold of.
Doesn't affect your hormones.
No prescription necessary.
Can be used while breastfeeding.

### Cons
People do worry about any negative side effects, but for most women, they're not a problem.

**The failure rate of using spermicide without a condom is pretty high, 29% for typical use, but it's better than using nothing at all.**

# Gazillions of Slang Words for Condoms

Back Pack
Bag Lady
Baggie
Banana Bandana
Banana Peel
Beanie My Cecil
Bobby Sock
Body Armor
Bone Blanket
Bone Bonnet
Boxing Glove
Bubble Boy
Bullet Casing
Candy Wrapper
Catholic Catheter
Chicken Charriot
Child Proof Lid
Cock Cap
Cock Cloak
Cock Frock
Condom
Corn Dog
Corn Husk
Crash Helmet
Cum Catcher
Cum Cup
Cumbrella
Cyclops Eye Patch
Dick C. Cup
Dick Dam
Dicktionary
DNA Lounge

Doggie Bag
Don Johnson
Dong Depot
Dong Sarong
Dork Cork
Driving Glove
Dunce Cap
Dust Cover
Emergency Brake
Filling Station
Fornication Filtration
French letter
Freudian Slip
Galloshes
Gent Tent
Glad Bag
Glove
Go Between
Goggles
Gonad Goggles
Hard Hat
Hatch Catcher
Haute Couture
He Stick Hindrance
Head Gasket
Head Light
Heaven's Gate
Hickory Dickory Dock
Hog Holster
Holds the Mayo
Hood Ornament
Hose Wrapping

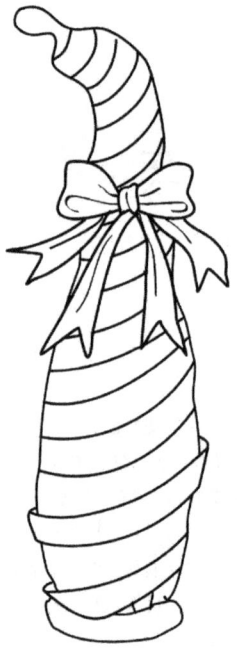

**Gift Wrap**

Hot Dog Bun
Hub Cap
Jack in the Box
Jewelry Box
Jimmy Hat
Jock Jacket
Juice Jar
Loin Luggage
Love Capsule
Love Glove
Love Shackle
Lover Cover
Luger Locker
Manhole Cover
Member Muzzle
Missile Mask
Mount Hood
Muzzle Loader
Nookie Nook
One-Eyed Beret
Parachute
Pen Top
Peter Pouch
Pillar Pullover
Pillowcase
Pit Stop
Pole Vault
Pony Stable
One-Eyed Willie's Eye Patch
Mr. Happy's Business Suit
Major Woody's Uniform
Little Red Riding Hood
John Thomas Overcoat

Pork Cork
Potatoe Skin
Pricknic Basket
Prophylactic
Pump Sump
Rain Fly
Raincoat
Rascal Wrapper
Restrictive Headgear
Rod Pod
Rubber Fence
Rubber Policeman
Safety Nut
Saran Wrap
Sausage Skin
Scabbard
Schlong Shed
Screw Top
Seat Belt
Sheath
Shower Cap
Shower Curtain
Shrink Wrap
Sleeve
Slug Housing
Snakeskin
Soup Bowl
Spanky Hanky
Sperm Bag
Sperm Dam
Sperm Worm
Sperminal Terminal
Spiral Binder

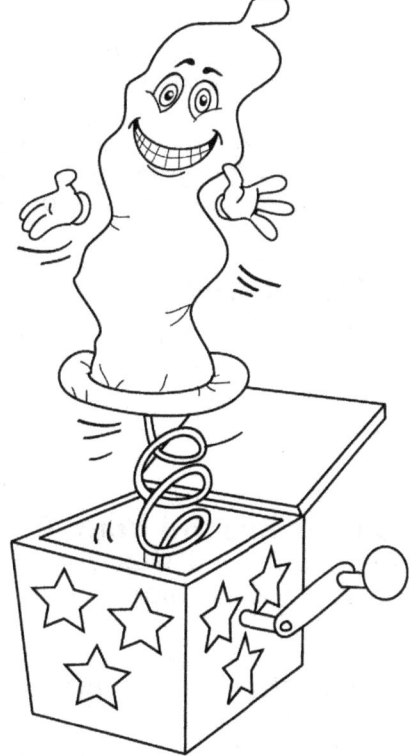

**Jack in the Box**

# Pubic Hair Facts

### Pubic Hair Protects Against Chafing During Sex
When one body rubs against another chafing may occur but pubic hair acts like a barrier and helps to protect and cushion the skin from being damaged.

### Pubic Hair Helps To Prevent Infection
Pubic hair can also protect the skin from potential bacteria and viruses. It helps to create microflora or helpful microbes because it absorbs sweat and keeps harmful particles from entering the vaginal area.

### Pubic Hair Turns Gray
Basically it behaves just as all the other hairs on your body do when you start piling on the years. It turns gray, thins out and sometimes even goes bald.

### Plucking Can Be Worse Than Waxing or Shaving
Waxing or shaving is better than plucking because plucking thick hairs particularly can be harmful to the skin. It can create more ingrown hairs that irritate or even increase the chance of infection.

### Pubic Hair Is Often A Different Color Than The Hair On Your Head
Your pubic hair is more likely to be the color of your eyebrows than the exact same color of your hair.

### Regrowing Pubic Hair Can Be Painful
Ingrown follicles can make the regrowth pubic hair uncomfortable, itchy and even very painful.

### Hair Removal Is More Painful Around Your Period
When is the least painful time to have a wax ? Well apparently it is less painful a week after your period when you have a higher pain threshold.

### Fancy Wearing A Merkin ?
Get this, Victorian ladies would shave their bits to prevent lice infestations for goodness sake ! The solution was a pubic hair wig or Mirkin worn over their vaginas. The female version is usually made of fur, beaver pelts or a soft cloth and they are still sometimes used for theatrical and movie scenes.

### Pubic Hair Souvenirs
During the 1700s and 1800s the British upper class had a dubious habit of collecting the pubic hairs of lovers as souvenirs almost like hunting trophies. Just to show their sexual prowess they would even attach them to their hats for all to see. No internet social sharing sites for this form of boasting yet, thankfully.

### The Record For The Longest Pubic Hair
The longest pubic hair to have ever been recorded belongs to a woman called Maoni Vi who lives in Cape Town, South Africa. The length of her pubes has been measured at an unbelievable 28 inches and that is just one of them. Imagine what the remaining bunch looks like !

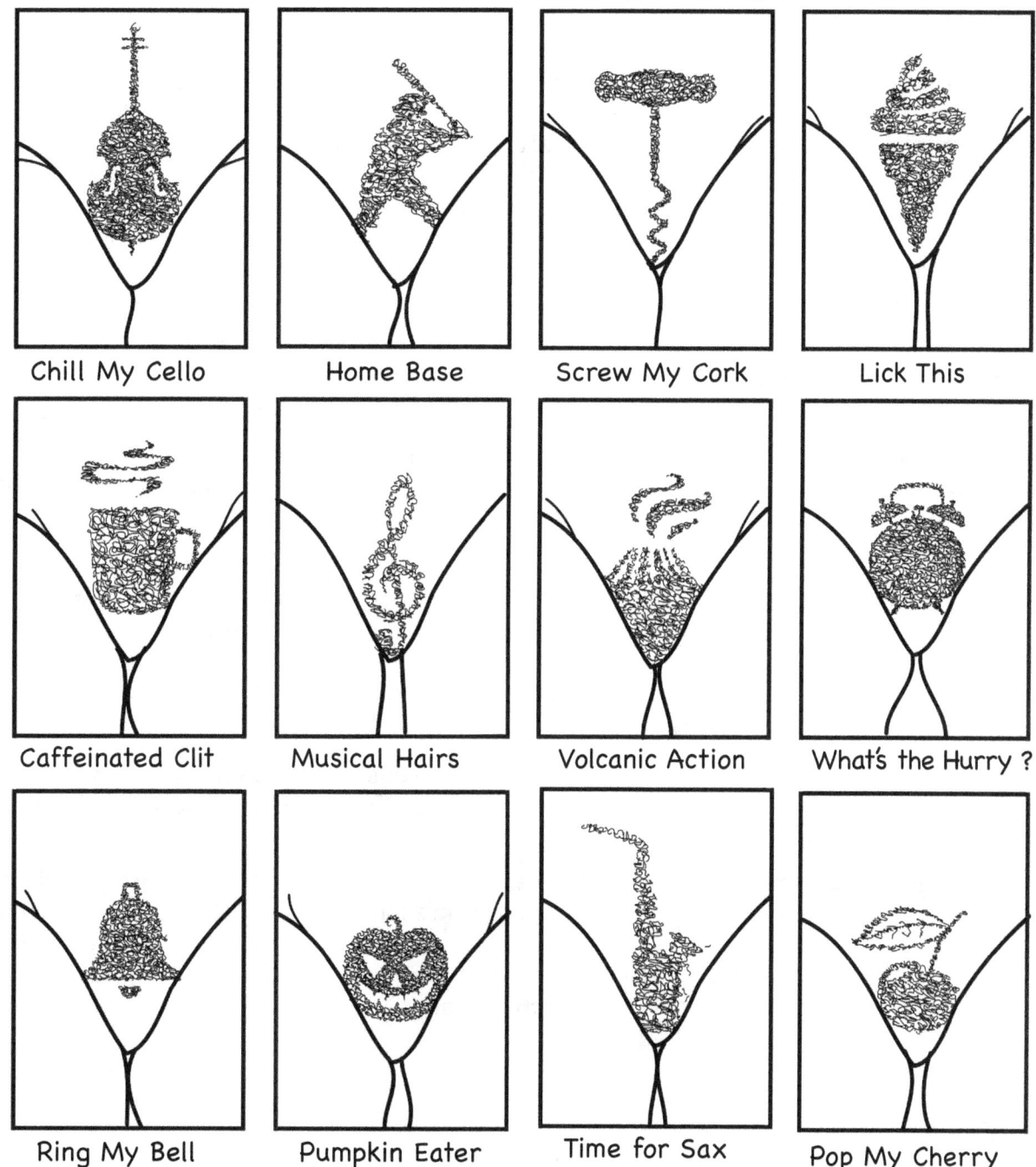

# Beware Vampire Pubic Crabs!
## CAUTION, IF YOU ARE SQUEAMISH DO NOT PROCEED!

This section should only be read at Halloween when sheer horror and awfulness is the name of the game. We all like wildlife of course but sometimes insect wildlife in particular can move into areas we really don't want them to. Such it is with the nasty little creatures called "Crab Louse" that look just like little crabs when viewed through a strong magnifying glass. They are wingless parasites of the most horrible and disgusting kind. They can under certain circumstances take up residence in our pubic hairs and at night they bury their heads inside pubic hair follicles and suck our blood. Not only that, our bodies can react to the proteins in their saliva bites and can become inflamed creating itching and red spots.

Does this horror story get worse? Well yes indeed. Infested children are at risk of lice spreading to their eyelashes, resulting in possible infections.

Unmitigated terror....Right? I told you. Creepy crawlies having a warm and cozy nightly haute cuisine at our expense. Yet another reason to keep our sexual relationships closely guarded. These critters are highly infective and are transmitted mostly through sexual contact.

Sexual contact is the not the only way to get them however. Even if there's no sexual penetration, you can get also crabs through skin-to-skin contact with someone who's infected. It is even possible to get pubic lice from wearing infested clothing, sleeping in an infested bed, or using contaminated towels or other linens. This is rare but it can happen.

So...what to do? How do we prevent these disgusting invaders from getting a foothold on our short and curlies and how do we control them? How do we make them stay away from our worst nightmares?

Unfortunately shaving the affected area, contrary to belief, will not eradicate either crabs or other STIs. Another common misconception is that pubic lice are spread easily by sitting on a toilet seats. This would be extremely rare. These lice cannot live far from a warm human body and they do not have feet designed to hold onto or walk on smooth surfaces such as toilet seats.

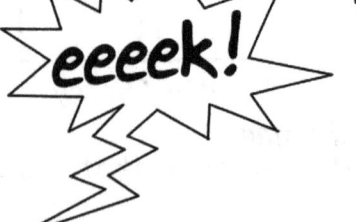

# Prevention and Control

The following are steps that can be taken to help prevent and control the spread of pubic ("crab") lice:

• All sexual contacts of the infested person should be examined. All those who are infested should be treated.

• Sexual contact between the infested person(s) and their sexual partner(s) should be avoided until all have been examined, treated as necessary, and re-evaluated to rule out persistent infestation.

• Machine wash and dry clothing worn and bedding used by the infested person in the hot water (at least 130°F) laundry cycle and the high heat drying cycle. Clothing and items that are not washable can be dry-cleaned OR sealed in a plastic bag and stored for 2 weeks.

• Do not share clothing, bedding, and towels used by an infested person.

• Do not use fumigant sprays or fogs; they are not necessary to control pubic ("crab") lice and can be toxic if inhaled or absorbed through the skin.

• Persons with pubic lice should be examined and treated for any other sexually transmitted diseases (STDs) that may be present.

CDC, Centers for Disease Control and Prevention. Department of Health & Social Services

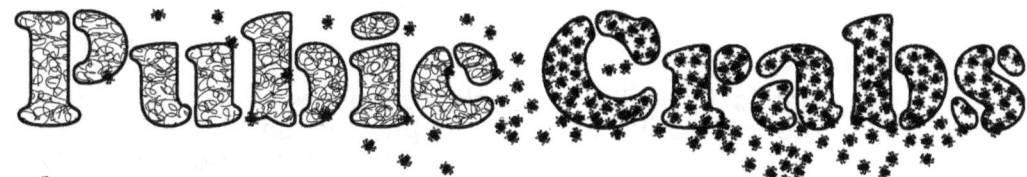

# Special Designer Condoms

There are many styles of condoms including, classic, ribbed, dotted and contoured but creativity has extended itself far beyond just the basic ones and even colored and flavored condoms are almost limitless in their variety.

### Glow in the Dark Condom
Love Light is a phosphorescent condom that glows in the dark. You will never get lost at night again. They do not shine brightly enough to find your way home in the dark so don't even think about it.

### Spray on Condom
A German firm has developed a spray-on condom tailor-made for all sizes. The liquid condom comes in an aerosol can that you spray onto the organ in question. A few seconds later, the liquid solidifies into the familiar latex and forms a tight seal. It's still in the testing phase so it might be a while before it hits the neighborhood drug store.

### Customized Condom
"MyFace Condoms" are FDA approved, lubricated condoms which are customizable to include your name, picture, special message or anything else you choose. Unfortunately, the images only appear on the condom wrapper instead of the actual condom which would be more entertaining.

### Condometric Condoms
Condometric is the only prophylactic that shows off the penis' length. It is printed with ink that won't cause an allergic reaction but still, it might create other unexpected reactions bordering from "Jeez" to hysterical laughter.

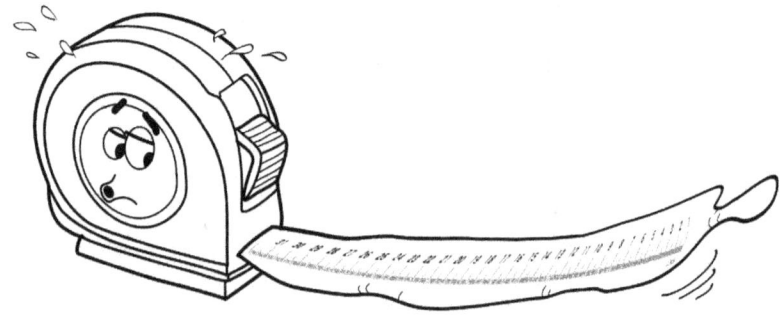

### Anti-Rape Condoms
Rapex is a device that is basically a female condom with teeth lining the inside that work just like the protective spikes in a parking garage. You can go in, but whatever you do, don't back out. The teeth are angled so they allow penetration, but bite like a shark as the penis is removed; supposedly causing so much pain that it will give the woman a chance to escape. Further, according to the designer, the device will need to be surgically removed at a hospital, which will help to lead to the capture of the rapist.

## Camo Condoms
Yes, there are even camo condoms hiding out there somewhere if you look hard enough !

## Smart Condom
The world's first 'smart condom' which rates a man's sexual performances and can detect STIs has been created by scientists.

The i-Con Smart Condom is billed as the newest form of wearable technology in the ever-growing market.Providing a range of statistics, including duration, speed and girth measurements, it enables users to even assess their sexual prowess. The device also records the amount of calories burnt, different positions and can detect chlamydia and syphilis.

## Dinosaur Condom
This dinosaur condom can actually be used as a condom although the producers don't guarantee you or anyone else in the vicinity will be fully protected from the sharp teeth.

## Tuxedo Condom
The only FDA approved printed condom available, this condom is appropriate when you want to be best dressed for the occasion which hopefully is not a costume party.

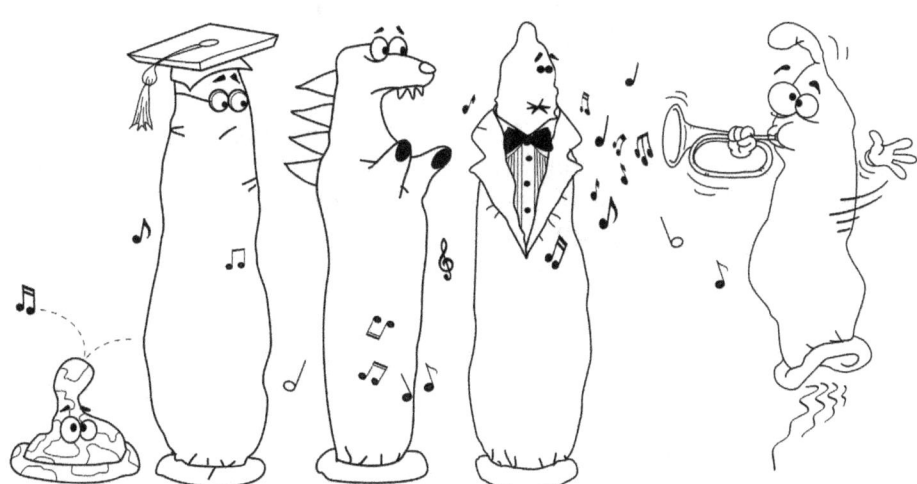

## Musical Condom
A man by the name of Hryhory Chausovsky, a scientist in Ukraine, claims to have invented a new type of condom that plays music during intercourse. Music volume depends on intensity of love-making and tone varies based on the sexual position and by forceful movements. So far there have been no attempts to create an orchestral piece to accompany this condom but one can be sure that eventually there will be one coming to a concert hall near you soon !

# Flavored Condoms

### Whiskey
"I followed my heart and it led me to whiskey."

### Pumpkin Spice
"Tomorrow is October, which means. the Great Pumpkin is Coming." Peanuts comic strip, Charles M.Schulz.

### Bacon
"It started the way so many good things do: with bacon." Paula Garner, Phantom Limbs

### Nutella
"All you need is love and a little bit of Nutella does not hurt." Ad slogan.

### Garlic
"Garlic is good to chew and fumigate." 8th Century BC Assyrian Health Guide. Ouch....!

### Soda
"It had to be good to get where it is." Soda slogan 1926.

### Cannabis
Cannabis supporters in the medical industry have long claimed that cannabis increases appetite for a lot of things, but they can't always remember what they are.

### Durian
Durian, or Green Hedgehog, is a fruit found in Southeast Asia that is so smelly it's banned on public transport in Singapore as well as certain hotels in Southeast Asia where it is considered the "King of Fruits". The smell of Durian has been described as similar to onions, turpentine, raw sewage and moldy old gym socks. Whew....!

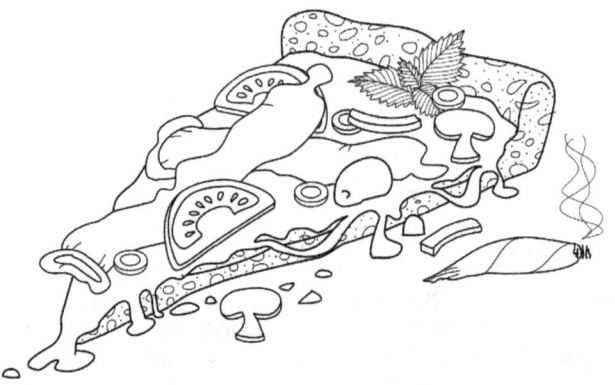

### Pizza
Russian Designer Marina Malygina combined pizza and safe sex by making condoms look hot out of the oven complete with their own individual boxes.

### Other Flavors

Menthol/Peppermint/Lemon/Banana/Orange/Grape/Strawberry/Vanilla/Blackcurrant/Cherry/Peach/Chocolate/Pineapple/Rose/Cocacola/Green apple/Tuttifruiti/Coffee.

# Curious Condom Facts

## The Thinnest Condoms in the World
Sagami rubbers boast a thickness of just .01 mm. The hairs on your head now have an average thickness of .06 mm. The condom is visible and it's completely safe, too. This newly released rubber has been tested over 200,000 times in the lab for quality assurance and has sold out in Tokyo since it hit the shelves.

## How Many Condoms Are Used Each Day ?
Roughly 14 million a day. 5 billion are sold each year. It is estimated that 13 billion are needed worldwide.
Around 87 condoms are used each second on Valentine's Day in the US. Valentine's Day really lives up to it's title of National Condom Day.
Total number of condoms sold in the U.S. each year. 450,000,000. Whew...

## What Countries Use The Most Condoms ?
Zimbabwe's condom usage now tops that of any other country in the world, with over 109 million condoms used in 2014. the British come in second, according to Australia-based Ansell. The United States ranks sixth.

## Condoms Used In Musical Theatre
Cats, was the first Broadway show to experiment with condoms to protect body microphone receivers from perspiration. As of 1997, the long running musical had reportedly used approximately 49,000 condoms on stage. No record of how many were used backstage.

## Discrete Condom Protective Cases
There are some really nifty condom cases that can be found online. They are cheap and unobtrusive in appearance. Much better than leaving one molding in your wallet for months getting more of a battering in it's wrapping than it would out of it.

## Great Sex With A Condom
If you're using the proper condom size and lube, the old excuse that "condoms don't feel good" does not apply. Surveys actually show that couples were just as satisfied with sex whether or not they were using condoms. Throw in the fact that condoms are 98% effective at preventing pregnancy and make sex ten-thousands of times safer, you really have no excuse not to wrap it up. Condom usage does NOT affect the quality of a woman's orgasm.

## Can Condoms Break ?

It can happen if they are not used correctly. Here are a few tips that make condoms even less likely to break.

Store condoms in a cool, dry place and not in your wallet or very tight pockets for Long periods of time. Check the expiration date to make sure the condoms you're using are still good.

Use water or silicon-based lube. Lube reduces the friction that can lead to breakage.

Make sure you put the condom on before you start having sex, and keep wearing it until you've finished and pulled out.

## What is a Condom's Shelf Life ?

Condoms have a shelf life of approximately 4 years, if it is not stuffed and getting stale in your wallet or purse that long.

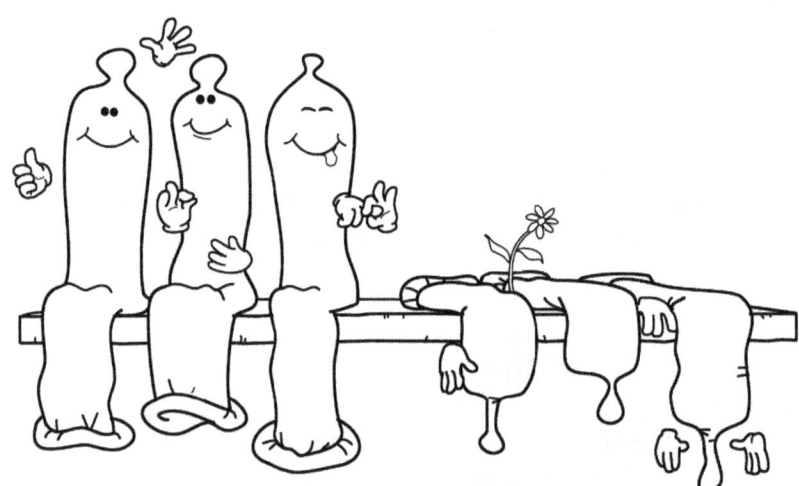

## What is the Longest Condom Chain ?

In case you have been wondering, there is even a Guinness World Record for the longest condom chain. The chain of condoms is 10,726 feet, six inches, and was achieved by Population Services International in Bucharest, Romania, in 2007. The chain was tied together by 1,683 participants with Love Plus condoms, a brand of the time that donated 100 percent of its sales to fund programs working to prevent HIV and AIDS.

# What are the World's Most Expensive Condoms ?

Safe sex comes at a price in Venezuela where abortion is illegal and rates of HIV infection and teenage pregnancy are among the highest in South America. Men are paying $650 for pack of 36 !

A 200 year old condom has been found to be the world's most expensive. Sold at a whopping $600 the 18th-19th century contraceptive isn't made from latex, but sheep intestine. I'm sure the sheep in question would be proud but suffering from acute indigestion if it were still around.

Naked's box of 6 luxury condoms cost $12.90.

# Where are Condoms Made ?

Asia is the center of the global condom network. Thailand leads world output at 3 billion condoms per year, exporting 12 percent of their capacity to the United States. (The U.S. no longer produces condoms on a large scale. The last major factory, located in Alabama, shut its doors after USAID stopped buying condoms for international AIDS prevention from the company in 2009.) The top five producing countries are all in Asia, with a combined annual total of 11.6 billion. Karex in Malasia is the world's largest producer of condoms. Iran is also getting into the act, with a state-funded factory producing 45 million condoms per year.

# How are Condoms Tested ?

Manufacturers put their products through a battery of quality tests. They hang up test condoms and fill them with water and stretch pieces of latex until they break and the even conduct "burst" testing by inflating the rubber like a balloon to see how much pressure it can handle. Manufacturers test every condom for pinholes by trying to pass an electrical current through the rubber. They even place a few samples in the oven for a week to accelerate the aging process, and run the tests all over again.

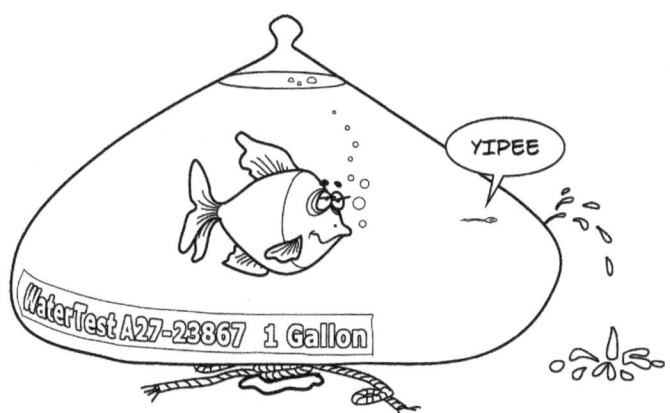

# Fun Condom Tips

## Start a Fire With One

Latex condoms can be ignited easily with an open flame, making a really good fire tinder. It will burn for several minutes, giving you enough time to build a fire.

## Fishing Bobber

A make-shift condom bobber is pretty darn effective. Thanks to a US trade embargo and the inefficiencies of Cuba's centrally-planned economy, thousands of products are near impossible to find on the island. This forces Cubans to make do with what they have, and condoms have been put to many new uses.

Dozens of fishermen inflate them and use them off Havana's seaside promenade, or Malecon, where these improvised bobbers carry bait far out to sea and increase its resistance against tugging fish.

## Carry Water In It

A condom can carry up to 2 liters of water but when used it as a water container, you have to give it some sort of support. When a condom is expanded and carrying water, it becomes very delicate and easily punctured so fill the condom that is placed inside of a sock which will give it some support. Note that you should still purify your water if it is stored in a condom.

## Survival Sling Shot

Use 3 unused condoms on each fork of a previously carved out pocket sized sling shot frame made from a natural tree fork. This will provide the force necessary to kill small game. Put the condoms inside each other with a little wad of cattail fuzz at the bottom and use duct tape to hold each condom band on the frame. Wrap the other end of the condoms around the loop of bank line and duct tape it in place.

More information is available online if you are having overwhelming survival issues and want to be prepared for just about everything.

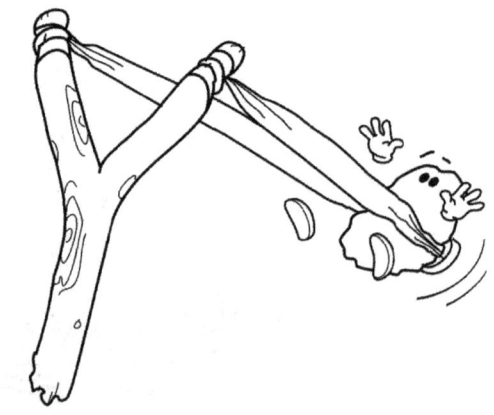

**Bear Trap Protection** ( A must do for all bears !)

Tony Black is a comedy hypnotist who tours colleges and performs at weddings. One of his latest stunts is to put his condom-clad hand into a bear trap. Tony an Irishman, pulled off the unusual stunt in a show called 'Dirty Trancing'. He pulled a condom over his hand and then bravely put his hand into the bear trap, allowing it to suddenly snap on his hand.

Incredibly, the condom appears to prevent the trap from breaking his skin, acting as a protective layer. The condom seems to provide enough protection for the trap to leave him unscathed.

This proves the amazing strength of a condoms as, without one, placing a hand or any penile implement inside such a trap and activating it would normally do a boat load lot of grimace producing damage.

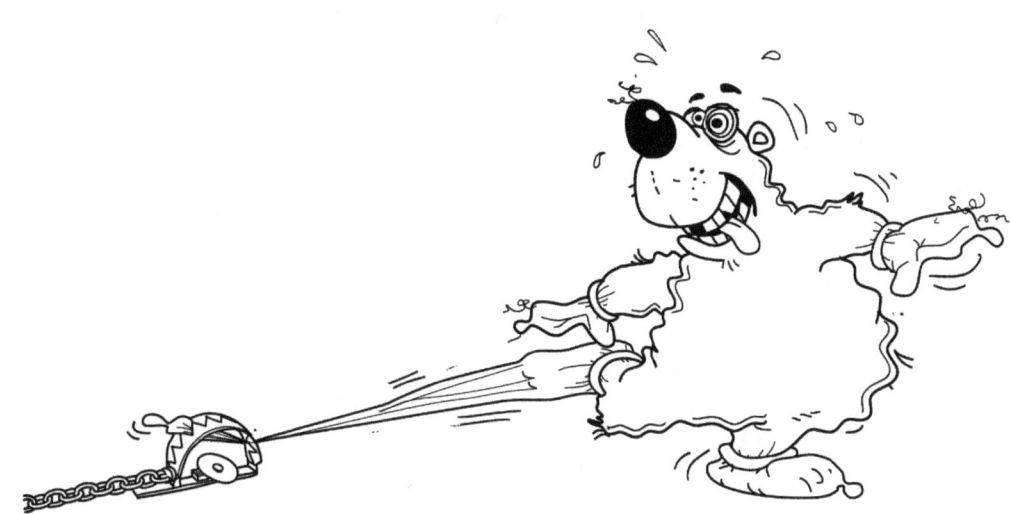

Bears of course will welcome this piece of good news but, unless back country adventurers are crawling around on all fours in bear country they won't ever have to use this unique type of protection that bruin now enjoys !

Just another novel use for condoms that makes the world a better place to live in, even for bears that would never normally think of utilizing discarded condoms to spare them the embarrassment and annoyance of being caught in a stupid bear trap.

*It is not recommended that you attempt this trick at home using one of your neighborhood kids or local marauding bears.

## Protect Your Muzzle
Cover the muzzle of a rifle to prevent sand/mud/water from getting inside is a very simple and effective technique for keeping everything clean. Discard the condom afterwards of course.

## First Aid
In a worse case scenario, a condom can be used as a crude surgical rubber glove while dealing with any first aid related issues. It will protect the wound as well as protect you from the wound if you're dealing with someone else.

## Elastic Bands
Slice up a condom horizontally to make individual and very useful elastic bands. Do not re-use the condom bands for contraceptive purposes once the condom has been sliced up as their their efficacy is now more than just a little bit suspect.

## Protecting Your Electronics
Condoms can stretch over most smartphones and other electronics. Tie it up tightly to make them waterproof maybe when you are on a rafting or sailing trip for instance.

## Galoshes
If you have a brand new pair of expensive leather shoes all shined up and ready to impress then use condoms to cover and protect them when you get caught in a nasty rainstorm and the side walks are covered in muddy puddles. Just remember to take them off before you slide into a full elevator on your way to a work interview on the 30 floor.

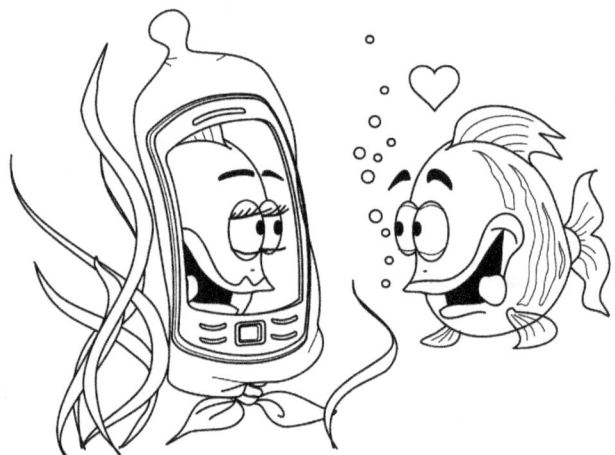

## Smoothing Out Roads
In India many of the hundreds of millions of condoms that are handed out each year never have a chance to enjoy the dirty deed. Instead they are mixed with tar and cement to create smoother more durable road surfaces.

## Vadge Condom Popsicles (A must have for all new mothers !)

Any new mother will tell you that giving birth can leave you in great pain long after the baby has been delivered. However, one new father has revealed the unconventional method he used to ease his partner's discomfort.

On the parenting site DAD Martin Wanless wrote that he used condoms filled with water and then frozen to help relieve post-birth soreness and swelling. An icy cold condom is the perfect shape to rest in between a new mum's legs and ease a bit of pain and swelling" he says. So, shortly after giving birth in hospital, his wife was presented to a fridge full of frozen condoms.

Martin isn't the only one to have relied on this inventive method to ease his wife's pain, certain midwives also recommending it as a pain reliever. Speaking to "Parents" Katie Page, a certified nurse-midwife in Lynchburg Virginia, said she often prescribes the frozen condom to new mothers. She said: 'Fill up a condom with water, tie the end and freeze it to make a tube of ice. Wrap it in a clean, cotton T-shirt. It fits really nicely against the perineum".

Apparently this method has also been recommended by other midwives as well but so far ice cream vendors have not yet decided to add these useful products to their range so you have to make them yourself.

Take care not to insert these into the vagina and make sure to avoid ice burns by not coming into direct skin contact with it. As a precaution always check with your midwife or health visitor before using this handy popsicle.

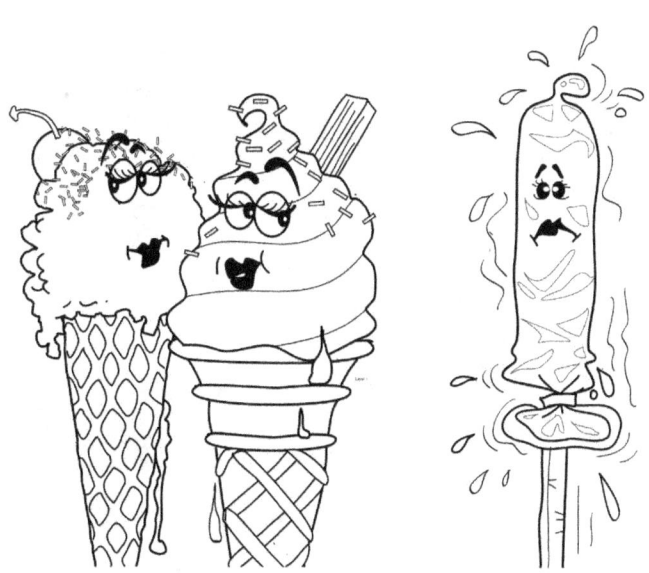

## Condom Vino

A US trade embargo and the inefficiencies of Cuba's centrally-planned economy, has made thousands of necessary products near-impossible to find on the island.

This forces Cubans to make do with what they have at their disposal and condoms have been put to many other uses even serving as condom fishing bobbers that are very popular and widely used to great effect.

Believe it or not the Cuban El Canal Winery, a flourishing business in Havana run by Orestes Estevez a tough-looking and very affable former Ministry of the Interior Official, has hundreds of bottles capped with condoms which slowly inflate as the fruity mix ferments and produces gases. They work as fermentation blocks.

When the fermentation is over and the gas is depleted the condom stops inflating and falls over all limp, the wine is ready for bottling.

'Putting a condom on a bottle is just like with a man. It stands up, the wine is ready, and then the process is completed,' Orestes says. Well almost completed anyway......a bit more attention may be required to make the process really complete.

## Haute Couture Condomwear

Going to the prom and can't think of anything glamourous to wear? Getting married and can't really afford a wedding dress ? Going to a costume party and need a nifty costume that will make everyone else seem under dressed ?

Well, now there is some great news for you that will solve your apparel problem every time.

Make your own exotic fashion statements by creating "condom wear" from colored condoms ! This is a new sexy fashion trend that is now on the rise in the fashion condom kingdom. Don't be caught with one's pants down, grab a boxful of colorful condoms and get to work designing great looking prom or wedding dresses, lingerie or even risqué bikinis for beachwear.

Your groom or date can rent an inflatable condom costume for any occasion and you will be a matching pair that will enthrall and delight the vicar, the congregation, the prom party, your grandparent's birthdays or even the attendees of a friend's baby shower. Go ahead, be adventurous and reveal your absolute sexy self by wearing this bodacious Haute Couture fashion wear statement. Wear these trendy costumes when you are out on the town or impress your neighbors by wearing them gardening in your back yard.

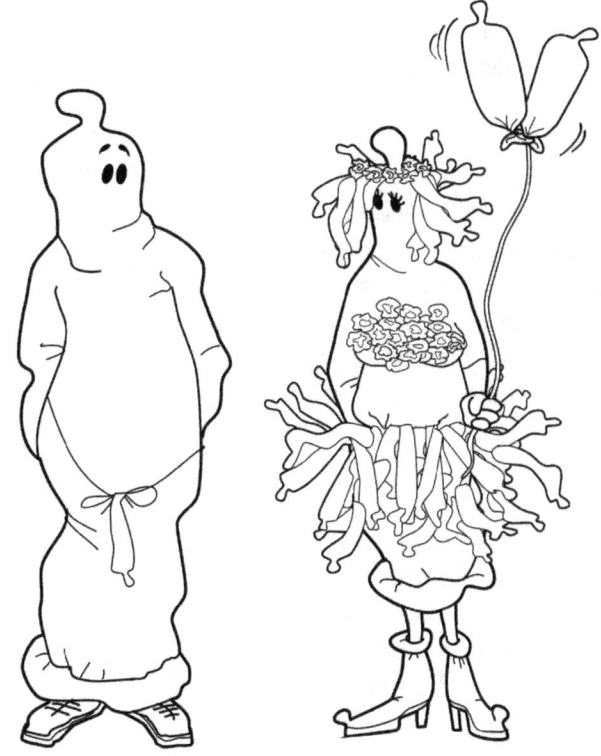

Check out all the splendiferous "designer condom events" that are happening at locations near you. These are are popular events used to promote HIV and safe sex awareness. International Condom Day, a February 13th holiday in conjunction with Valentines Day, an event promoted by AHF and it's global partners, is celebrated in 65 cities in more than 25 countries around the world.

# Foreign Words for Condoms

## European

Albanian - prezervativ
Basque - kondoia
Belarusian - прэзерватыў
Bosnian - kondom
Bulgarian - презерватив
Catalan - condó
Croatian - kondom
Czech - kondom
Danish - kondom
Dutch - condoom
Estonian - kondoom
Finnish - kondomi
French - préservatif
Galician - preservativo
German - Kondom
Greek - προφυλακτικό (profylaktikó)
Hungarian - óvszer
Icelandic - Smokk
Irish - coiscín
Italian - preservativo
Latvian - prezervatīvs
Lithuanian - prezervatyvas
Macedonian - кондом
Maltese - kondom
Norwegian - kondom
Polish - prezerwatywa
Portuguese - preservativo
Romanian - prezervativ
Russian - презерватив (prezervativ)
Serbian - кондом (kondom)
Slovak - kondóm
Slovenian - kondom
Spanish - condón
Swedish - kondom
Ukrainian - презерватив (prezervatyv)
Yiddish - קאָנדאָם

## Asian

Armenian - պահպանակներ
Azerbaijani - qandon
Bengali - কনডম
Chinese Simplified - 避孕套 (bìyùn tào)
Chinese Traditional - 避孕套 (bìyùn tào)
Georgian - პრეზერვატივი
Gujarati - કૉન્ડોમ
Hindi - कंडोम
Hmong - hnab looj
Japanese - コンドーム
Kannada - ಕಾಂಡೋಮ್
Kazakh - презерватив
Khmer - ស្រោមអនាម័យ
Korean - 콘돔 (kondom)
Lao - ຖົງອະນາໄມ
Malayalam - കോണ്ടം
Marathi - कंडोम
Mongolian - бэлгэвч
Myanmar (Burmese) - ကွန်ဒုံး
Nepali - कंडोम
Sinhala - කොන්ඩම්
Tajik - рифола
Tamil - ஆணுறை
Telugu - కండోమ్
Thai - ถุงยาง
Urdu - کنڈوم
Uzbek - prezervativ

## Other

Esperanto - kondomon
Haitian Creole - kapòt
Latin - condom

## Austronesian

Cebuano - condom
Filipino - kondom
Indonesian - kondom
Javanese - kondom
Malagasy - fimailo
Malay - kondom
Maori - ure

## African

Afrikaans - kondoom
Chichewa - kondomu
Hausa - kwaroron roba
Igbo - condom
Sesotho - khohlopo
Somali - cinjirka
Swahili - kondomu
Yoruba - kondomu
Zulu - ikhondomu

## Middle Eastern

Arabic - واق ذكري (waq dhikri)
Hebrew - קוֹנדוֹם
Persian - کاندوم
Turkish - prezervatif

# List of Elite Condom Reservoir Patrons

1. Baby Batter
2. Ball Barf
3. Bonkjuice
4. Buttermilk
5. Choad Nectar
6. Clam Sauce
7. Cock Droplets
8. Cock Snot
9. Cough Drops
10. Cuckoo Spit
11. Crack Wax
12. Cream
13. Crud
14. Cum
15. Custard
16. Daddy Sauce
17. Dongwater
18. Erectoplasm
19. Face Cream
20. Fish Dip
21. Flour Water
22. Fructis
23. Fun Gel
24. Gentleman's Relish
25. Glue
26. Happy Trails
27. Hemulsion
28. High Fructose Porn Syrup
29. Honey
30. Hot Milk
31. Jam
32. Jamba Juice
33. Jazz
34. Jelly
35. Jizz
36. Layonnaise
37. Letch Water
38. Liquid Silk
39. Live Cultures
40. Load
41. Love Liquor
42. Male Tears
43. Man Chowder
44. Man Foam
45. Man Period
46. Man Seed
47. Monkey Juice
48. Nobslurry
49. Nizzle-Drizzle
50. Nut Butter
51. Oil of Man
52. Oil of Ulay
53. Ointment
54. Onward Christian Soldiers
55. Oyster Droppings
56. Pale Marmalade
57. Pearl Jam
58. Penis Colada
59. Pole Milk
60. Population Paste
61. Prick Liquid
62. Protein Shake
63. Pube Solvent
64. Pudding
65. Rude Glue
66. Salad Dressing
67. Satchel Syrup
68. Schlong Jelly
69. Scum
70. Sink Bubbles
71. Slime
72. Snake Spray
73. Soap
74. Spaff
75. Spendings
76. Spew
77. Splashback
78. Splooge/Spooge
79. Spratz
80. Spume
81. Spunk
82. Squiggle
83. String of Pearls
84. Tadpoles
85. Tail Juice
86. Tallow
87. Throat Yogurt
88. Trouser Gravy
89. Turkey Spit
90. Wad
91. Wang Pus
92. Wank Paste
93. Weiner Sauce
94. Wet Paint
95. White Gold
96. White Honey
97. White Light/White Heat
98. White Ribbon
99. Willymilk
100. Wormgob

# Is Finger Length Linked to Penis Size ?

Guys: Hold up your right hand. According to Korean researchers if your index and ring fingers are mismatched, congratulations, you're more likely than men with matching digits to be endowed with a longer schlong dongadoodle.

Prenatal testosterone may in part explain the differences in adult penile length. Men who have relatively long ring fingers are thought to have been exposed to high levels of testosterone in utero, and this has been linked to aggression, athleticism, sexuality and intelligence.

Digit ratios are non invasive and easy to measure so, when a possible flame closely inspects and then grabs a man's hand while producing a tape measure it may be an indication that they are contemplating some kind of future festive frolicking of the intimate kind.

## Measuring Digit Ratio

Use a ruler of calipers to measure the distance from the middle of the bottom crease to the tip of the finger. Once you have the measures for both your ring and index finger, then divide the length of your index finger by the length of your ring finger. The result is 2D:4D (2nd digit divided

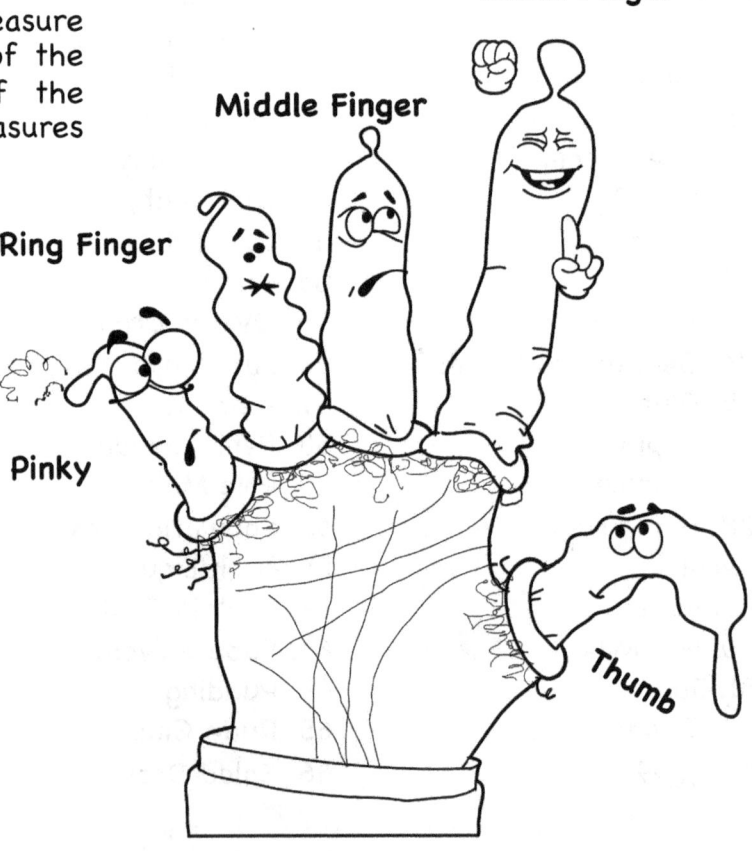

**N.B.**
Wearing gloves to avoid detection when you go on a new dinner date is not recommended.

# Eye Watering Male Privates in The Animal Kingdom

## Average Penis Sizes of Various Animals

Blue Whale : 120 inches
African Bull Elephants : 78 Inches
Giraffe : 48 Inches
Bull : 30 Inches
Barnacle : 25-50 Inches
Walrus : 25 inches
Rhinoceros : 24 Inches
Tapir : 19 Inches.
Roberto Cabrera : 18 inches
Pig : 18 inches
Argentine blue-bill lake duck : 17 inches
Stallion : 12-18 Inches
Green Sea Turtle : 12 Inches
Hyena : 7 Inches.
Banana Slug : 6-9 Inches

**Average Human : 5.56 inches**
Chimpanzee : 3 inches
Gorilla : 1 inch
Shrew : 1/5th Inch
Bee : 1/10 thousands of an Inch
Men in one study had members that ranged from 1.6 inches long to 10.2 inches long.

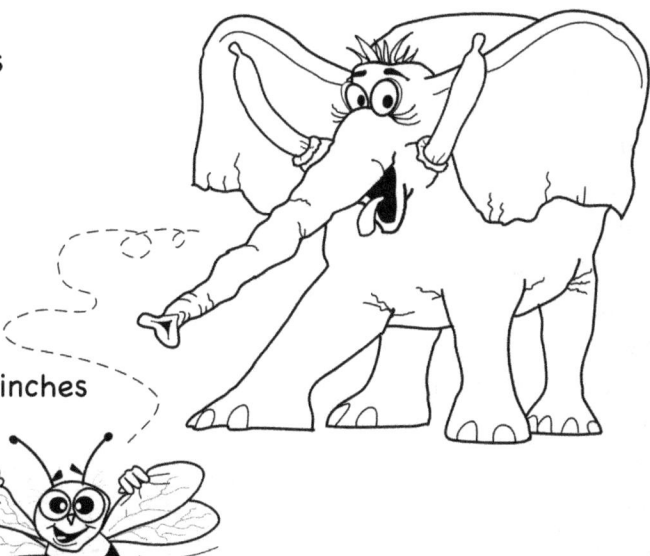
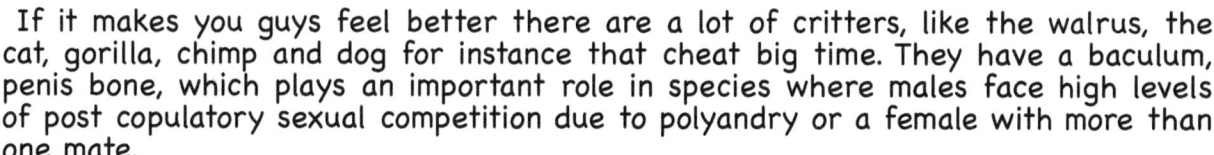

If it makes you guys feel better there are a lot of critters, like the walrus, the cat, gorilla, chimp and dog for instance that cheat big time. They have a baculum, penis bone, which plays an important role in species where males face high levels of post copulatory sexual competition due to polyandry or a female with more than one mate.

## Penile Spines

These are exactly what they sound like: small spines on the head of the penis of many animals. There are plenty of animals that sport the spikes, including a type of nasty beetle called the bean weevil whose hard, sharp spikes scar the female beetle's reproductive tract during sperm delivery. Many rodents, primates, such as marmosets, and even pythons whose Y-shaped hemipenis is often spined in order to grip the walls of the female's opening, known as a cloaca. There is a key molecular switch from a key gene that's required to form the spine and, thankfully for the ladies, humans trashed it a long time ago.

# Fancy Names for Fancy Parts

There are hundreds of fancy part names, here are just a few for your delectation.

**Dude Parts**
Albino Cave Dweller
The Artful Throbber
Bell on a Pole
Burrito
Chopper
Don Cypriano
Custard launcher
Dickie
Ding Dong McDork
Dude Piston
Eggroll
Giggle Stick
John Thomas
Krull The Warrior King
Little Elvis
Love Stick
Meat Popsicle
Microphone
One-Eyed Trouser-Snake
Pig Skin Bus
Plonker
Ramburglar
Schlong Dongadoodle
Schmeckel
The Bone Ranger
Tallywhacker
Todger
Tool
Trouser Snake
Whoopie Stick
Wiener Schnitzel
Wing Dang Doodle
Winkie

**Dudette Parts**
Cooch
Whisker Biscuit
Honey Pot
Rattlesnake Canyon
Fuzz Box
Love Rug
Vadge
Wizard's Sleeve
Grassy Knoll
Curly Curtains
Cupid's Cupboard
Sugar Basin
Silk Igloo
Golden Palace
Yo Yo Smuggler
Clamarama
Jelly roll
Hairy Heaven
Feld of Dreams
Tinker Bell
Wolly Bolly
Ponchita
Cha Cha
Dildo Hotel
Candy Kiss
The Big Casino
Coochie Pop
Panty Hamster
Cupid's Cupboard
Holiest of Holies
Toolshed
Petticoat Lane
Quim

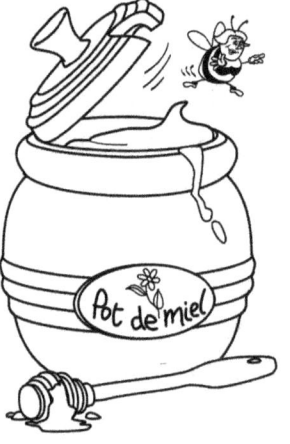

**Honey Pot**

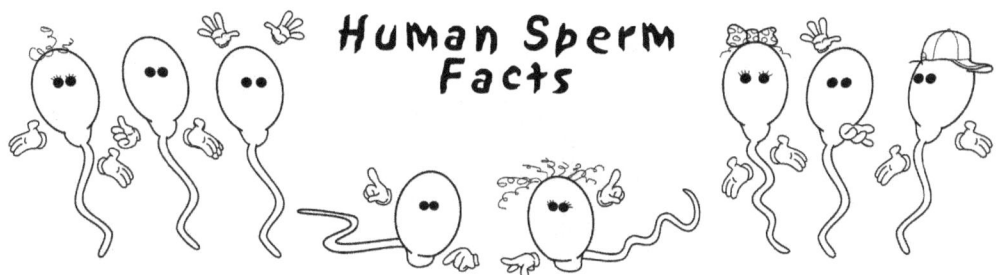

# Human Sperm Facts

### What is sperm made of ?
Semen only contains about 10% sperm - the rest consists of enzymes, vitamin C, calcium, protein, sodium, zinc, citric acid and fructose sugar. A sperm is the smallest cell in the human body. A human egg is the largest but who's boasting ?

### How many are there in a male ?
A healthy male produces about 70-150 million sperm a day - but when you ejaculate, you can lose 3 times that ! Sometimes, if they don't disappear entirely, it can take hours to find out where they all went, which is why it's better to round them all up in a condom reservoir right from the outset. It sure saves checking out the ceilings and walls for any errant spaff.

### How long do they live ?
When inside a woman's body, a sperm can live up to 5 days without sending out an SOS for help and assistance.

### What sex are they ?
There are male and female sperm - the females are slower, but stronger, while the males are faster, but weaker. Nature, in it's wisdom, thinks of everything.

### How many are released at one go ?
Average volume of semen per ejaculation is 1 teaspoon which equates to about 200-500 million of those little guys in the average amount of semen produced each time you release.

### How fast do they move when released ?
The average speed of semen at the moment of ejaculation is 31 mph but only if there isn't a nasty headwind to slow them down.

### How far can they travel ?
The human male ejaculates on average distance of 7 to 10 inches, the world record for the farthest spoof is 18 feet!

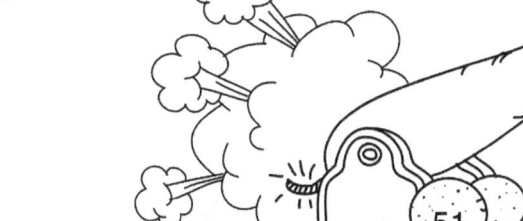

# Human Egg Facts

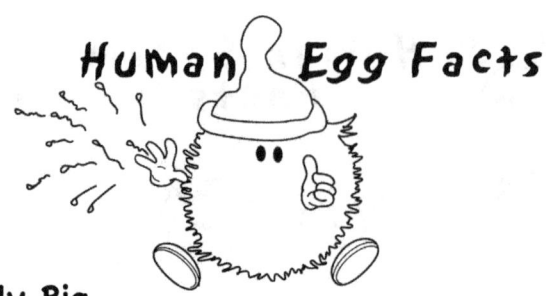

## A Human Egg is Really Big
The human egg is the largest cells in a woman's body and no other cell in the human body is anywhere near that big. It is about the size of a grain of sand. (Sperm cells are the smallest human cells. They are no more than a nucleus with a small amount of cytoplasm, some mitochondria and a long tail. More sperm cells are released during a single ejaculation than a woman produces in her entire life.)

## A Woman's Eggs Take a Long Time to Mature
Most eggs are present within the ovary in an immature state from the time of a woman's menarche. A few eggs will lie dormant for years or even decades before they begin to fully mature. For eggs to complete their journey to ovulation, they must receive a signal to begin their final maturation process about 150 days before they are released from the ovary. At the beginning of any given cycle there may around 12 eggs that have started to grow, and as ovulation nears preference is given to one of those eggs and as it receives the final push to maturity it is then released from the ovary.

## The Egg Has a Short Life After Ovulation
Once the egg has matured and is released from the ovary during ovulation, it goes into the fallopian tube where it lives for 12 to 24 hours. Conception is possible if sperm is already present in the fallopian tubes when the egg is released, or if a woman has sex while the egg is alive, causing sperm to swim up through the uterus and into the fallopian tube. Sperm can reach the egg in as little as 30 minutes. If conception is successful, the newly fertilized egg will travel out of the fallopian tube and implant into the uterus 6 to 10 days later. If the egg is not fertilized, it will simply dissolve and pass out with the menstrual flow. Though the egg has a lifespan of less than a day, sperm can stay alive inside a woman's uterus and fallopian tubes anywhere from 1 to 5 days. This means that sex up to 5 days prior to ovulation can actually result in pregnancy!

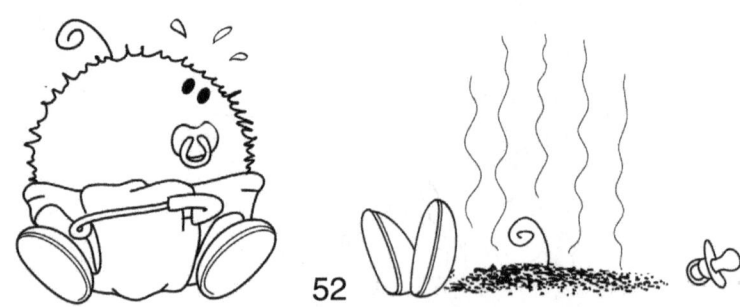

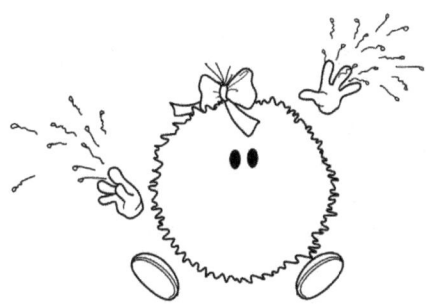

## Healthy Eggs

Young women have plenty of healthy eggs and about 90 percent of the eggs of a 21-year-old woman are viable. Alas, only about 10 percent of the eggs of a 41-year-old woman might be viable which is why young women are having their eggs extracted and frozen just in case they choose to have babies later on in life.

## Multiple Ovulation

Multiple ovulation is the release of two or more mature eggs during a cycle. This is said to occur in up to 10 % of all cycles which means that an average woman releases two or even more eggs per year. When two eggs are released and both are fertilized it results in fraternal twins. Identical twins, however, are produced when a single embryo is split into two.

When double ovulation occurs it happens as part of a single ovulatory event and the eggs will be released within 24 hours. Once ovulation occurs a big hormonal shift takes place, progesterone production is revved up and the release of any future eggs is prevented.

## Picky Eggs

Eggs can even be picky. We usually think of the sperm as doing all the work of fertilization when it penetrates an egg but it is now believed that it is the egg that chooses which sperm is admitted, or not.

Apparently the egg appears to prefer sperm with intact DNA and in doing so produces a compound that softens the outer layer of the egg to allow the lucky sperm to enter.

Recent studies suggest that the egg amy actively bind the sperm to it's surface leaving the sperm with no choice in the matter. Once this happens the egg hardensand any further entry by other sperm is prevented.

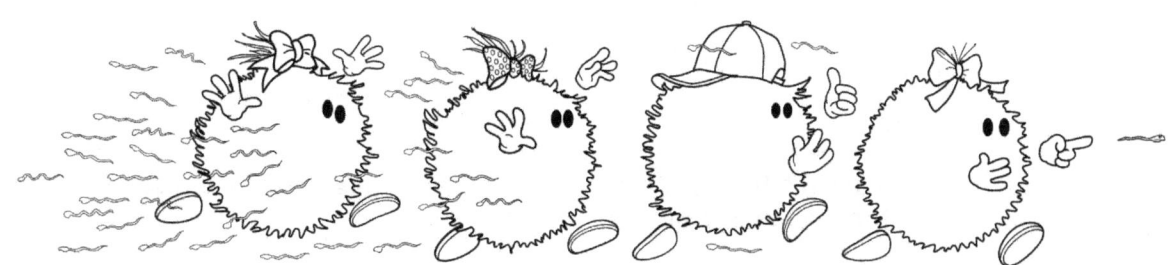

# Showers or Growers ?

Are you, or is your man, a "**shower** or **grower** ?" Well, if it makes a bloke feel better, approximately 71% of men are growers.

The difference between growers and showers is partly genetic and partly to do with a man's health. There are medical issues that cause dysfunction such as diabetes and cardiovascular diseases.

Flaccid penile length doesn't correlate with erect penile length. What does correlate with erect penile length is a penis put on full stretch. Grab hold of your penis and pull it as hard as you can as if you're trying to pull it off. The propensity of the penis to grow is directly proportional to how far you can pull it away from the body.

The coefficient of penile linear expansion describes how the size of a manly appendage changes with the ambient temperature. This rule of thumb also depends on genetics, health and a certain amount of luck.

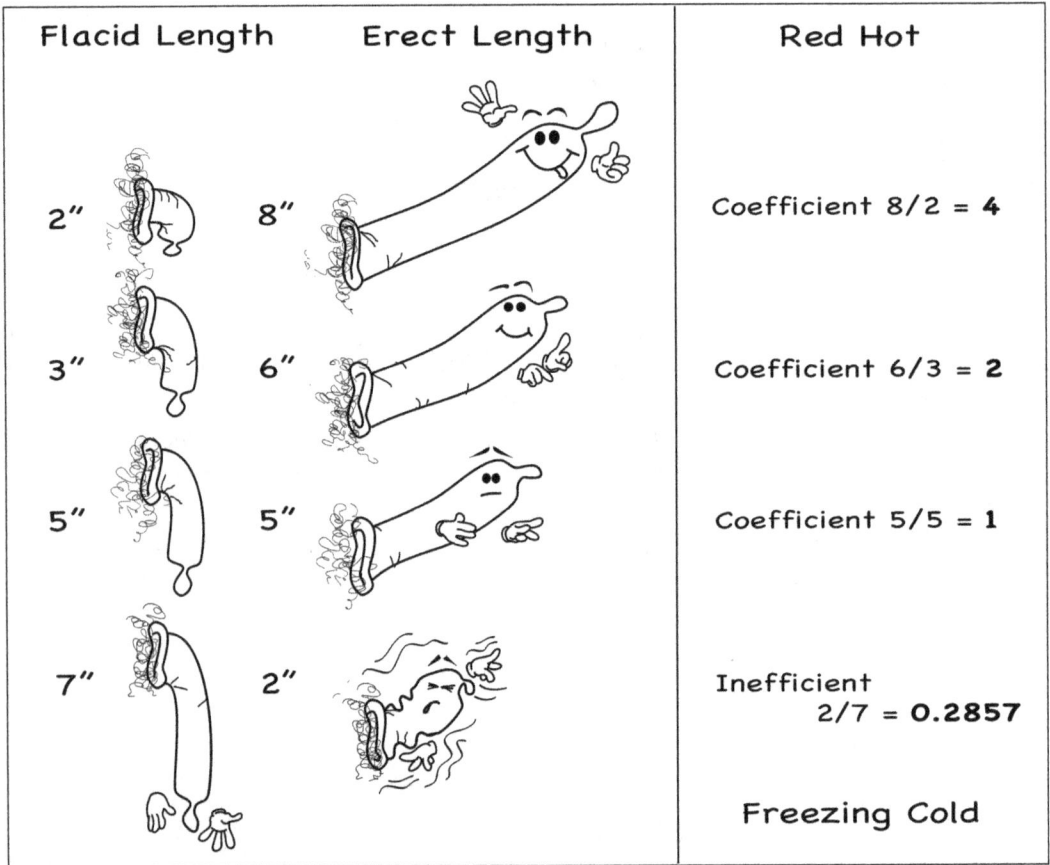

**The linear coefficient rule of thumb fails miserably when member is exposed to minus degree temperatures for prolonged periods of time !**

# Erectile Disfunction/Impotence

Occurs when a man can't get or keep an erection firm enough for sexual intercourse. Useful facts for those who are unable to do more with a condom than just color one !

More than 3 million US cases per year.
Treatable by a medical professional.
Usually self-diagnosable.
Lab tests or imaging rarely required.
Chronic: can last for years or be lifelong.
Erectile dysfunction can be a sign of a physical or psychological condition. It can cause stress, relationship strain, and low self-confidence.

Patients suffering from erectile dysfunction should first be evaluated for any underlying physical and psychological conditions. If treatment of the underlying conditions doesn't help, medications and assistive devices, such as pumps, can be prescribed.

## Ages affected

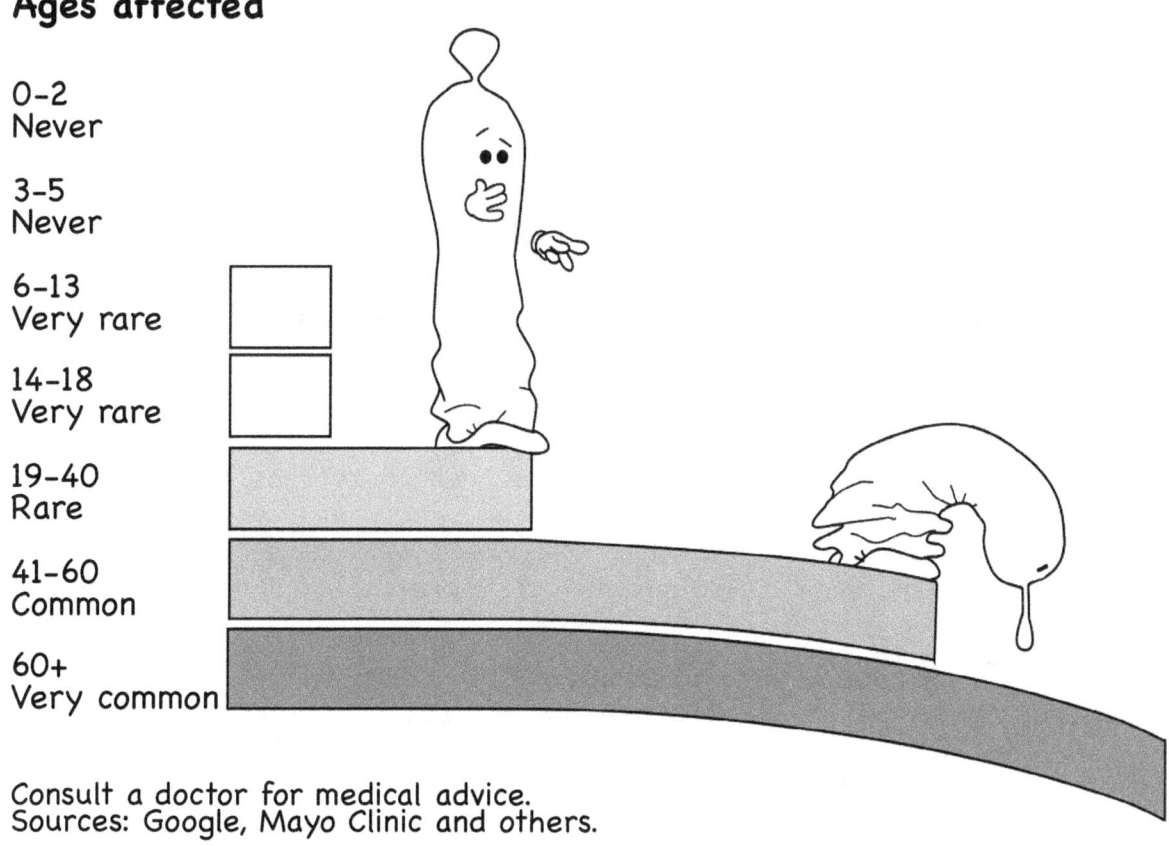

0-2
Never

3-5
Never

6-13
Very rare

14-18
Very rare

19-40
Rare

41-60
Common

60+
Very common

Consult a doctor for medical advice.
Sources: Google, Mayo Clinic and others.

# Strange Forms of Ancient Birth Control

Don't like condoms? Then consider for a moment what historical alternatives that were available to those that wanted to avert pregnancy. These rather ingenious techniques probably had a very spotty success rate and some were even dangerous and could potentially kill you but they are surprising in their absurdity or creativity whatever you want to call it.

## Moonshine

Once upon a time, in Greenland, the natives really believed that the moon and the moonbeams made women pregnant. The best way to avoid this was not to look at the moon and, just in case, rub magic spit on their bellies when they went to sleep. Sleeping on their bellies was another technique to avoid being impregnated although if they really wanted to actually get pregnant undressing under a full moon was the best way to make it work. "The moonbeams must have done it" may well be the best and most creative excuse for a guilty lover ever.

## Blacksmith Water

This was an idea that persisted from the ancient Greeks to World War I. Drinking blacksmith water which contained lead was thought to prevent pregnancy. However the exposure to lead can cause other health problems far worse than an unintended pregnancy like pain in the joints, nausea or vomiting, learning disabilities, fatigue and loss of appetite as well as irritability and hyperactivity.

## Weasel Testicles

A magical solution to ward off pregnancy, conjured up in the Dark Ages, was manifested in women wearing amulets that were created from weasel testicles. I have a feeling that it warded of a lot of the local weasels besides just the sperm.

## Lemons and Vinegar

This method of contraception dates back to the Talmud. How about using a sea sponge dipped in vinegar that has to be applied within seconds after sex or it might provide an even faster access to the cervix. Lemon juice was also a sponge option because it was thought that citric acid would work as a spermicide. As a side note, old Cassanova himself used lemon rinds to prevent pregnancy.

## Urine

The Middle Ages introduced an interesting idea for birth control and it involved wolf urine. If a women had sex and peed in the same spot that she-wolf had already peed she would not get pregnant. Strangely today's birth control pills are made from the urine of pregnant horses after the estrogen is extracted. Maybe this was because horses would stay still in a field and wolves would just keep running off to have private, instead of public, pees.

## Lace
Not to be confused with Hemlock, which is very similar and extremely poisonous the consumption of Queen Anne's Lace seeds were thought to be yet another form of birth control. The seeds, which are known as wild carrot, were eaten immediately after having sex and although the results were neither guaranteed or safe this belief has lasted from the fourth and third centuries BC until modern times.

## Lysol
There was a time when birth control was actually illegal in the US so what was the alternative of choice ? In the 1900s Lysol was advertised to women as a safe way to control their feminine hygiene and fertility when used as a douche. However it caused inflammation and burning and in later years almost 200 poisonings and even five deaths were recorded.

## Mercury
How about swigging a mixture of oil and mercury on an empty stomach ? The ancient Chinese used this trick to prevent unwanted pregnancy but because mercury is toxic to the human body repeated ingestion by a woman can eventually lead to infertility which is maybe why they thought it was a good idea.

## Honey
In ancient Egypt women coated their cervix with a mixture of honey and crocodile poop to prevent sperm from entering it and, lets face it, the poop addition would definitely make the sperm think twice before proceeding. Women that want to avoid synthetic hormones and chemicals can still use the modern version today which is a diaphragm coated with and stored in honey.

## Silphium
Meanwhile, in Ancient Greece and later ancient Rome there was a big demand for a now extinct plant called silphium which just about fulfilled every use imaginable. Apparently it worked as poison antidote, a perfume, a leprosy cure, hair treatment and yes even as a form of contraceptive as well. It was so popular and so treasured it eventually became extinct in the only place on the planet that it would grow, in Libya.

## Pennyroyal
This perennial creeping herb that kills germs, keeps insects away, treats skin diseases, venomous bites and mouth sores. It is also a cat and dog flea repellent and as a fragrance for detergents, perfumes, and soaps. Ancient Greeks and Romans used it to induce menstruation and abortion and a 1st century physician Dioscorides' mentions it was used as a birth control device as well, although drinking too much as a tea will kill you.

# Peyronie Problem

Some men have a bent penis for a harmless reason, the tubes inside are different lengths. These two tubes, called the corpora cavernosa, fill up with blood to create an erection. They can be different sizes which can create a curve shape in the penis but this is less obvious when it is flaccid. The penis can curve upwards, downwards or bent to one side.

As you get older the skin gets looser and the curve can look more pronounced. A curve which is a significant bend may also be a sign of Peyronie's disease which is estimated to affect up to 7% of males. The cause of this disease is not fully understood although it is thought that injuries to the organ may be involved. Scar tissue may form in a haphazard way which may create a nodule that can be felt. If it comes on slowly with no recollection of previous trauma researchers suspect that it may be related to genes. Peyronie's disease may cause problems getting or maintaining an erection (erectile dysfunction). Your penis may also become shorter as well.

A recent study by researchers in Texas, a team from Baylor College in Houston, linked this with various cancers.

One and a half million men in the study found Peyronie's disease brought on a higher risk of testicular cancer by 40 %, stomach cancer by 40 % and melanoma by 29 %.

It is now suggested that Peyronie's sufferers should be monitored for symptoms including scar tissue, erection problems and pain with or without an erection.

There are more than 200,000 US cases a year so it is quite common.

If symptoms are severe or worsen over time, medication or surgery is recommended.

Source Mayo Clinic and Others.

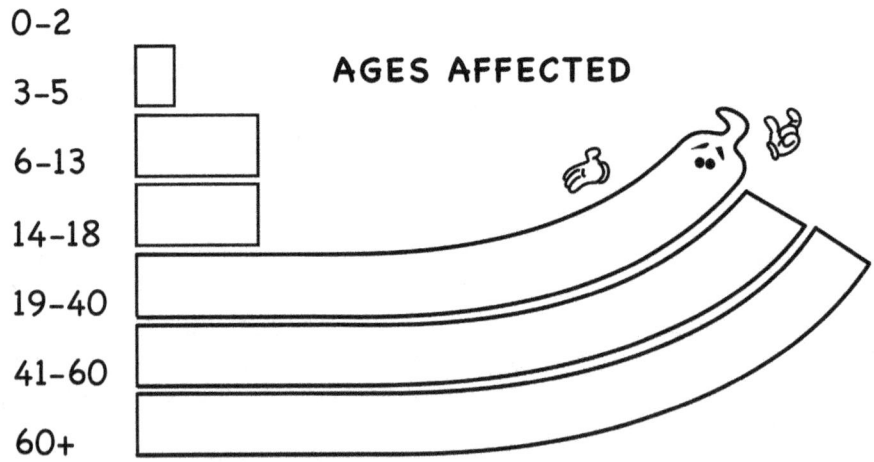

# Risky Sex

If you don't want to be all "creeped out"......read no further. This section is very creepy and is all about the Praying Mantis....a creepy critter with even creepier sexual predilections.

During sex, some female praying mantises have a tendency to kill their partners with a decapitating cutting blow to the neck.

This usually happens at the courting stage which is when males of all species really lose their heads but usually not so completely.

What remains of the male mantis continues to "get it on" as if the inclusion of it's head didn't really make a whole lot of difference to the task at hand. Like the horny insectoid zombie it is, the male continues to mate with the female, mounting her and delivering the sperm that will fertilize her eggs.

Apparently the male's body is still being controlled by nerves in its abdomen, and the Mantis "can still get the job done" without a head.

Believe it or not this is not done out of nastiness or spite or even an horrific random act of sheer unmitigated brutality. As a study by the State University of New York Fredonia tells us, males who get consumed by their mates are actually at a reproductive advantage. From a "selfish gene" perspective, this is actually good news for the amorous mantis and I'll bet he would be delighted to know this, if he still had the means to carefully consider it at length.

The female though, knows what she is doing. If they consume their partners they are able to reproduce twice the number of eggs than those who don't. I suspect that any male that survives probably loses their enthusiasm for mating and becomes celibate for the rest of their short but rather perilous existence.

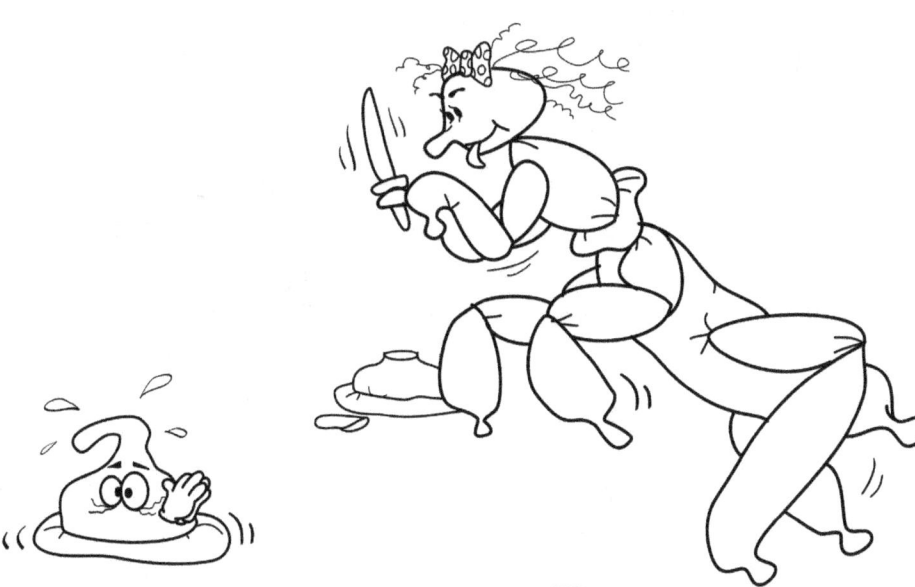

# "Stiffy" Slang

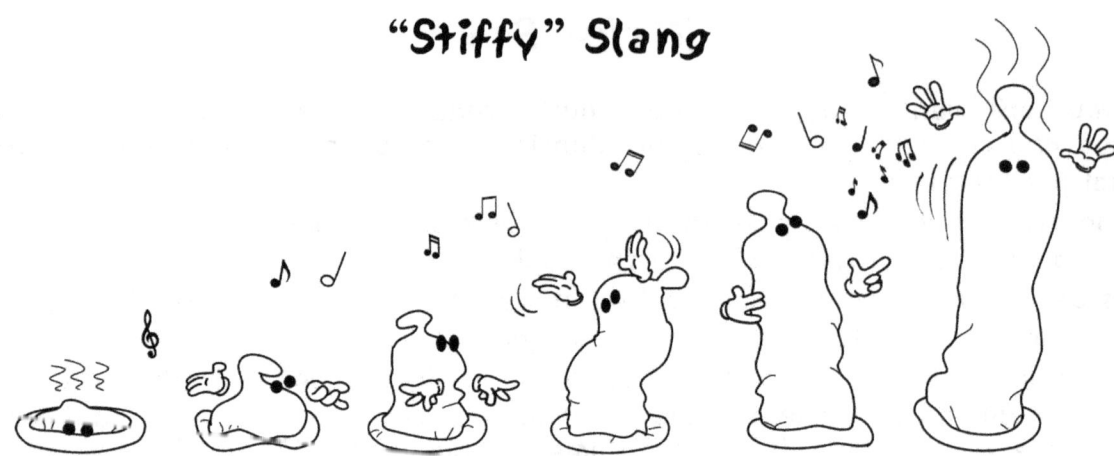

Throbbing Member
Officer at Attention
Angle on your Dangle
Boner
Homo Erectus
Cracked a Fatty
Stub Chub
Woody
Hard On
Pokey
Pitch a Tent
Woodrow
Meat Wrench
Thrill Drill
Vlad the Impaler
One Hole Friction Whistle
One Hit Wonder
Hellraiser
Vagina Miner
Bone Daddy
Morning Glory
Throbbing Gristle
Pocket Rocket
Custard Launcher
Full Salute

Purple Headed Yogurt Slinger
Wang
Baby Batter Blaster
One-Eyed Trouser Snake
Love Pump
Blue Veined Junket Pump
Salami/Sausage/Pepperoni
Snow Cannon
Lap Rocket
Raging Salmon
Goop Shooter
Fun Gun Mammoth Mountain
Bone-a-Phone
Pan Handle
Blue Steel
Cushion Pusher
Skroink Master
Pork Sword
Moby Dick
Happy Gilmore
Rodney
Longy
Goo Geyser
One-Eyed Muscle
Boney Baloney

Cock-a-Saurus Rex
Chicksicle
Dr. Feelgood
The Early Riser
Easy Rider
Elmer the Glue Shooter
The Impregnator
Jerkin Gherkin
Joystick
Long Dong Silver
Love Torpedo
One-Eyed Milkman
Pleasure Piston
Prince Everhard
Shiny Banana
Sergeant Stiffy
Skin Flute
Stretch Johnson
Spurt Reynolds
Taco Warmer
Sperminator
Super Soaker
Dick Sticker
Love Stick
Funky Fatty

# Wet Dreams and Flooding Nightmares

A nocturnal emission, commonly known as a "wet dream", is a spontaneous orgasm during sleep that includes ejaculation for a male, or vaginal wetness or an orgasm (or both) for a female. Dream emissions are most common during adolescence and early young adulthood, but they may happen any time after puberty and sometimes they occur into adulthood.

The possibility of potential wet dreams is not the kind of event usually included with the evening weather forecast so you never quite know exactly when to be prepared for them. Usually, wet dreams happen when you have a dream about sex rather than a dream about scoring a conversion while playing a winning game of professional football or tidying up your bedroom for the first time in two years.

Wet dreams are a normal part of growing up. There's nothing you can do to control or stop wet dreams. During puberty they are very common but once you start releasing sperm by masturbating or having sex with a partner, you may have fewer wet dreams and you will be relieved that your bed will once again return to just being an ordinary bed, instead of a bath tub.

If getting all wet and sticky when you sleep fills you with trepidation and you don't quite know when a wet dream may happen next, as a precaution, just take all the necessary steps to be as fully prepared as you can for a worse case scenario, in extreme cases, a flooding nightmare.

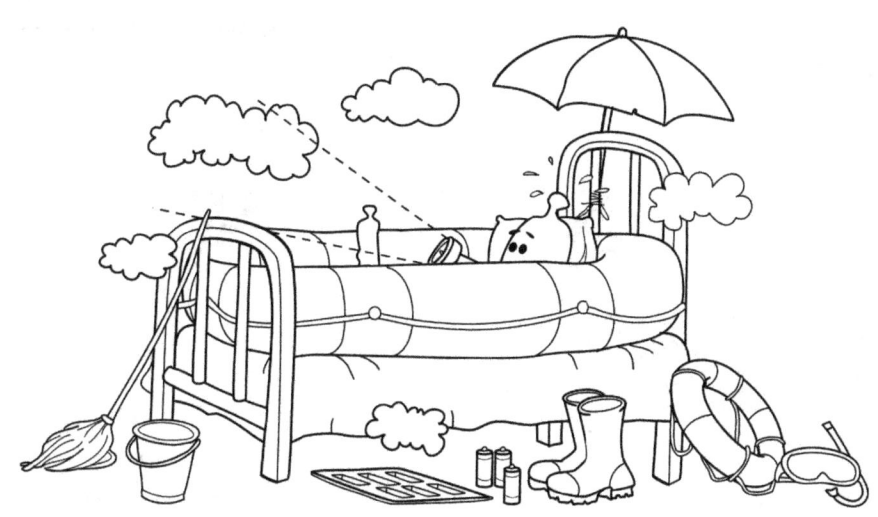

# Penis Park South Korea

There is a park called Haeshindang Park in a little village of Sinnam near Samcheok in South Korea that is dedicated to dozens of huge sculpted wooden and stone phalluses, some of them as much as 10 feet in length. There is even a fence made from penis shaped posts, penis shaped canons and a yawning man with a phallus emerging from his mouth.

These phalluses pop up like cram packed helmeted soldiers scattered all over a hillside, some straight up, some reclining and some every which way. They appear as totem poles, wind chimes, hollowed out benches with armrests and some are shaped like tortoises with penis heads sticking out from their shells. Some of the sculptured phalluses have smiling or scowling faces and added shaped limbs. There is even a group of realistically sculptured dudes fully dressed in Korean attire just standing around in a group letting it all hang out. Alas, there is no sign of a condom sculpture anywhere.

So how did this very popular tourist spot come into being you may ask ?

No-one knows quite when this park came into being but, according to legend (and South Korea's official tourism website) this was because of a nasty curse. A young maid was caught in a storm while harvesting seaweed and unfortunately drowned sitting on a rock when the awful weather prevented anyone from rescuing her. The fish stocks dried up and the villagers believed that the only way to get them back in their nets would be to appease the maid's spirit with male genitalia.

Other versions of the tale say that the locals figured out the connection between the need for phallic offerings and an abundance of fish when one of the fishermen relieved himself in the sea and the fish returned. To rid the town of this curse, giant penis sculptures were erected. Some people even believe it helps to satiate the virgin's inability to consummate her marriage. Will this remedy to such critical curses catch on whenever there is fishing problem in the world's fisheries? I guess. we'll have to wait and see.

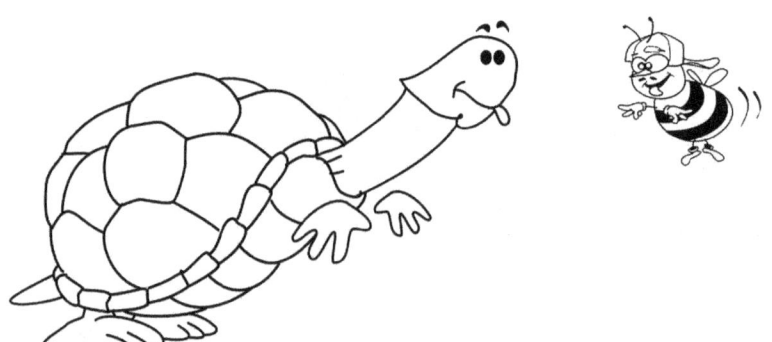

Haeshindang Park even has a tortoise sculpture with a penis head sticking out from it's shell.

# Phallological Museum Iceland

Meanwhile, at the other end of the world, Sigurður Hjartarson became the founder of the Icelandic Phallological Museum which now resides in Reykjavik. It is now one of Reykjavik's top tourist attractions and in 2011 had 12,000 visitors, 60% of them women. This Museum is probably the only museum in the world to contain a collection of phallic specimens belonging to all the various types of mammal found in a single country.

Sigurður started out in 1974 when a 'pizzle', a bull's penis, was presented to him while he was on a summer vacation in the countryside. It was used as a whip for animals. Some of his school teachers also worked in a nearby whaling station and they would bring him whale penises, supposedly, to tease him. By 1980 he had collected 13 species, four from whales and nine from land animals.

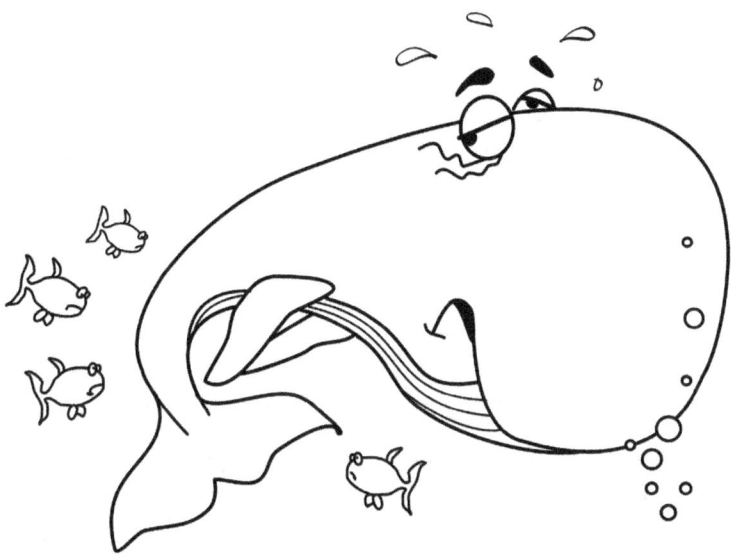

Now, there are more than two hundred penises and penile parts belonging to almost all the land and sea mammals that can be found in Iceland. This amounts to 282 specimens from 93 different species of animals. In the biological section there is a collection of 350 oddments and practical utensils related to the museum's theme.

Hjartarson's son Hjörtur Gísli Sigurðsson took over as curator in late 2011 and moved the museum from a small fishing village called Húsavík to Reykjavík where he has brought the display to a new more modernized level. He is now expected to set the standard for phallology worldwide.

# What Makes a Good Lover?

**What makes a truly great Male Lover?**
Here is a shortlist that will fulfill every woman's needs and desires.

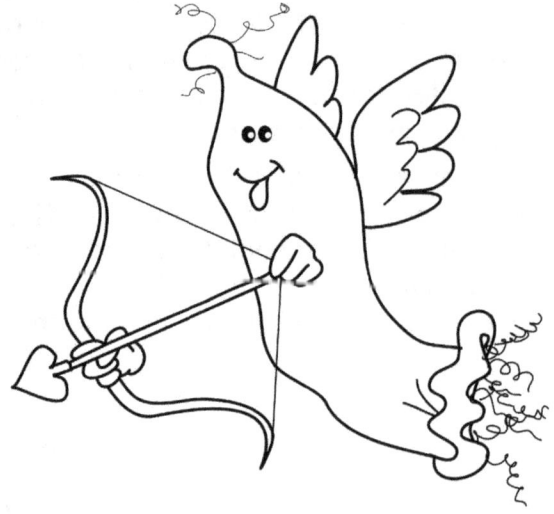

Make her feel sexy.
Listen to her.
Compliment her.
Maintain constant desire.
Be kind. Make her feel safe.
Show generosity.
Be ambitious.
Be trustworthy.
Keep a cool head.
Cultivate your masculinity.
Don't be judgmental.
Be innovative.
Be experimental.
Stay fit and healthy.
Be playful and passionate.
Be confident.
Be supportive.
Be spontaneous.
Be self deprecating.
Be a willing learner.
Be playful and passionate.

**What makes a truly great Female Lover?**
Here is a shortlist that will fulfill every man's needs and desires.

**(Apart from including every suggestion listed above, here are a few more to consider.)**

Don't call him a fat slob.
Don't tell him he never listens.
Don't hog the remote.
Don't tell him his friends suck.
Don't tell him he's always honky and needs a shower.
Don't tell him to mow the lawn in the middle of an exciting football game.
Don't tell him to stop picking his nose and start picking up his mess instead.
Don't call him an ignorant SOB.
Do scratch his back when asked.
Do pour him a beer without asking and while you are at it an oil change and lube on the family car would be quite nice too.

# World's Best Lovers

There have been numerous studies done over the years to determine which country has the best male lovers. A few of them are shown here and probably should be taken with a huge grain of salt.

Travel the world and test them out if you must but please do not be offended if the nationality of you or your lover is on the worst lover list.

## RANKED BY ENGLAND Study 2012

| BEST | WORST |
|---|---|
| 1- English | 1- Germans |
| 2- British | 2- Spanish |
| 3- Liechtensteiners | 3- Scots |
| 4- Outer Mongolians | 4- French |
| 5- Cameroonians | 5- Saxons |
| 6- I-Kiribati | 6- Danes |
| 7- Inner Mongolians | 7- Jutes |
| 8- Ni-Vanuatu | 8- Normans |
| 9- Mosotho | 9- Romans |
| 10-Caulkheads | 10- Vikings |

## RANKED BY AMERICA Study 2014

| BEST | WORST |
|---|---|
| 1- Americans | 1- Russians |
| 2- Texans | 2- Spanish |
| 3- Kyrgyz | 3- Italians |
| 4- French | 4- French |
| 5- Australians | 5- Australians |
| 6- Forgot | 6- Gibraltarians |
| 7- Germans | 7- Germans |
| 8- Irish | 8- Irish |
| 9- Maltese | 9- Mexicans |
| 10- Portuguese | 10-British |

## RANKED BY FRANCE Study 2013

| BEST | WORST |
|---|---|
| 1- French | 1- Germans |
| 2- French | 2- English |
| 3- French | 3- Germans |
| 4- French | 4- Dutch |
| 5- French | 5- Americans |
| 6- French | 6- Greeks |
| 7- French | 7- Germans |
| 8- French | 8- Scots |
| 9- French | 9- Turks |
| 10-Travaille toujours dessus | 10- Russians |

## RANKED BY GERMANY Study 2014

| BEST | WORST |
|---|---|
| 1- Germans | 1- French |
| 2- Germans | 2- English |
| 3- Hannah Schneider | 3- Swedes |
| 4- Norwegians | 4- Dutch |
| 5- Irish | 5- French |
| 6- South Africans | 6- Greek |
| 7- Australians | 7- Welsh |
| 8- Kiwis | 8- Scots |
| 9- Danes | 9- Czech |
| 10-Canadians | 10- Frau Meyer |

Among the reason given for the worst and the most horrible are... Too smelly, too lazy, too quick, too dominating, too rough, too lovey dovey, too selfish, too loud, too sweaty and too hairy. Reasons for the best are not mentioned but national pride probably has something to do with the results.

# Perfect Music for Quickies

**Love Vs Time** a short Romantic Piano Instrumental which lasts all of 26 seconds by composer Jongzijun is about the fastest love making music in existence. When the Flight of the Bumblebee is way too long for a quick roll in the hay then this works well for a Delicious Quickie but be warned as there is almost no time to get your condom on so plan ahead.

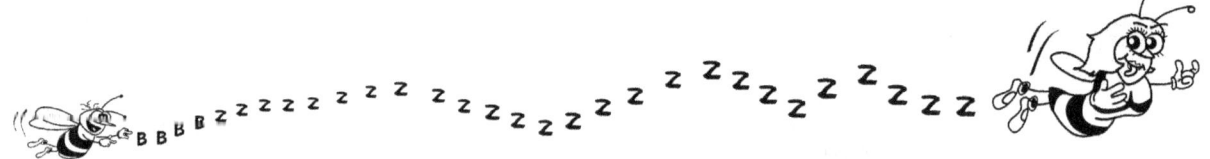

**Flight of the Bumblebee** is a famous classical piece written by Nikolai Rimsky-Korsakov .... Fastest performance for a good buzz. Oliver Lewis, a violinist, managed to play the piece in one minute and 3.356 seconds. Your Honey will love every short second of the flight but it is recommended that you should keep your safety belts on at all times in case of severe turbulence. Just enough time to get the condom in place and if you are really quick two and a half sexual positions are just about possible without reaching for the fire extinguisher.

**Ravel's Bolero** is a seductive piece of music, slow smoldering and hypnotic in the beginning but gradually building to a rousing crescendo at the end. If used to maximum advantage, one should expect at least three neighbor complaints as well as a possible visit from the local Fire Brigade. Lasts around 10 to 15 minutes depending on which orchestra is performing it. With a bit of dexterity and fortitude there is just enough time to squeeze in every page of the Kama Sutra except the Appendix page and the front and back covers.

**"Always Look on the Bright Side Of Life"** by Monty Python is a guaranteed antidote that will invoke positive feelings about any unfortunate love making disaster. This jolly track lasts for 3 minutes 58 seconds which leaves more than long enough time to put a smile back on anyone's face no matter how much disappointment and frustration they are feeling about the first 15 seconds.

**Rolling Stones "I Can't Get No Satisfaction"** is a great post track to play after an unsatisfying coitus adventure that doesn't quite arrive at the grand finale crescendo event one was hoping for. Three Minutes 55 seconds of pure self rightuous indignation, hopelessness and complete despair.

**"Keystone Cops Chase"** Silent Film Music. Yet another breathless two minutes 43 seconds of fast moving love making piano music for amorous oldies that miss the romance of a long gone B & W "fillum" era and wish to re-capture those distant memories of rapid paced passion in the back seats of the old Silent Movie cinemas. Check with your doctor and, just in case, arrange to have an ambulance standing by outside the cinema before pressing the "start" button if you can find it.

**"1812 Overture Full, with Cannons"** by Tchaikovsky. A very enthralling 15 minutes or so known for it's climatic volley of canon fire, ringing chimes and brass fanfare finale. Great lovemaking music but could be a bit risky indulging in the "naughties" during an out door Tchaikovsky concert. Bending over a cannon when they are fired can produce explosive climaxes but can also cause severe burns and loss of hearing. This reckless instance of supreme Tomfoolery is definitely not recommended for randy old pensioners who could easily lose their falsies, or more, to the heavens and even beyond.

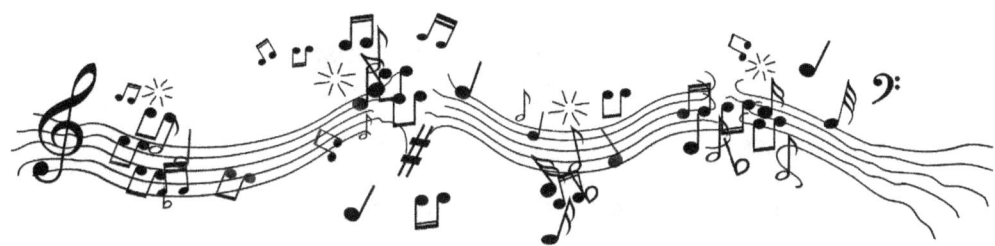

If for any reason you can't finish your business simultaneously to the very last note played in the above suggestions then set your sound system to "repeat" for as many times as you need to complete the job. For those that have a real challenge catching up with the pace of the music, set an alarm to go off in 30-45 seconds after you commence.

Of course, if you don't have to catch the train to work, take the kids to school, mow the lawn, take the dogs for a walk, do the laundry, clean the house, go grocery shopping, make dinner and put the trash out there is a great selection of romantic music available that lasts for hours and hours that will more than satisfy your endurance and love making requirements.

# Slower and Longer Romantic Playlist

OK time to get really serious and slow things down just a little bit. Maybe you do have plenty of time on your hands and you need specialized music that will transport you light years away to places in the Universe you have never imagined existed. Here are just a few selections to get you off to a slow start.

"No Ordinary Love" - Sade - 8 minutes 5 seconds...A voice like butter, like no other.....oozes sensuality with every note. Any Sade song will do the trick just nicely.

"J'taime" - Jane Birkin et Serge Gainsbourg - 4 minutes 20 seconds "Why does the French language sounds so sexy?" Breathlessly seductive as only the French can make it, which still works even after all these years.

"Sexual Healing," - Marvin Gaye - 4 minutes 06 seconds OK, it doesn't take long to be fully healed with this romantic masterpiece but you might want to make sure by being healed more than just once just in case the problem doesn't immediately go away.

"Can't get enough of Your Love Baby" - Barry White - 4 minutes 35 seconds Barry's surely the man for serving up luscious love making tunes that will keep you going all night long, which should be enough for anyone over 65 years old.

"Love Never Felt So Good,"- Michael Jackson and Justin Timberlake -4 minutes 07 seconds. Good recommendation for lots of loving.

"You Don't Know My Name"- Alicia Keys - 6 minutes 07 seconds A big laugh if it's a quick pick up and you are not even introduced yet but are already under the covers. ! Get introduced during the seductive phone chat section.

"Turn Me On" - Norah Jones - 3 minutes 53 seconds Romantic lyrics to turn you on......and on and on..............

"Ride On A White Horse " - Goldfrapp - 3 minutes 21 seconds Good beat for the galloping intervals, get the spurs ready for this one.

"A Whiter Shade of Pale " - Annie Lennox - 5 minutes 19 seconds Who cares about the miller and the nonsensical lyrics ? Annie's velvet seductive voice, the luscious backing and the sublimely slow pace makes this a winner every time.

"Sadeness" - Enigma - 7 minutes 37 seconds Mesmerizing and ethereal. Like making love on an alter during a church choir practice.

"Slow Motion " - Trey Songz - 4 minutes Not real slow but slow enough for most sessions.

'The Very Thought of You' - Natalie Cole - 4 minutes 17 seconds   Old time pure style and elegance with a simply gorgeous voice to melt your heartstrings.

"Night" - Robin Trower - 3 minutes 57 seconds   A magical and soulful and interstellar journey with Robin transporting us with his beautiful psychedelic blues tones. Dreamy and mystical, as is all his music.

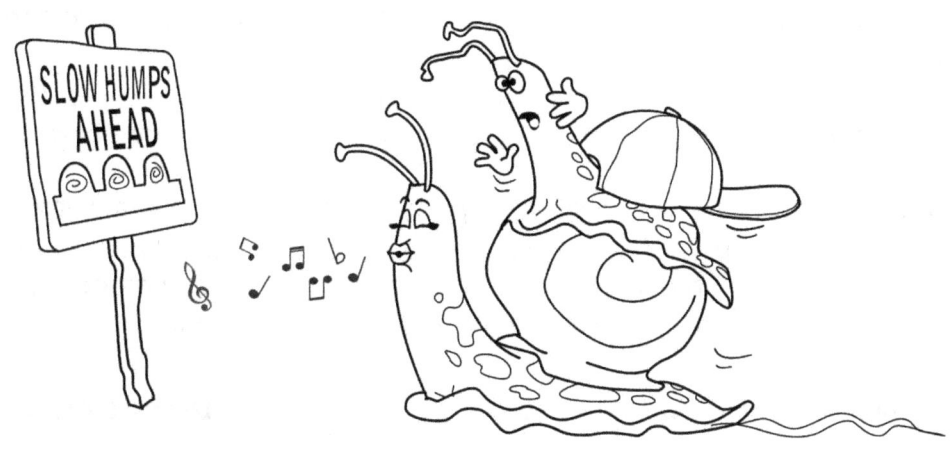

"Exotique " - Soul Ballet - 4 minutes 8 seconds   Heavy breathing in the liquid background that can only match the heavy breathing in the scintillating foreground.

"The Bedroom Best R&B 90's Sexy Love Music" - 55 minutes 33 secondS   To put you in the right mood for each and every minute.

"Dance for You" - Beyoncé - 5 minutes 14 seconds. Seductive and forceful as well as dreamy and playful.

"Earned It" From The "Fifty Shades Of Grey" Soundtrack - 4 minutes 35 seconds. Mesmerizing and ethereal, perfect for adding some extra color hues to your rainbows of euphoria.

"One More Light" -Linkin Park - 4 minutes 30 seconds.   Wistful and distant, RIP Chester. Thanks for making it happen.

"Let Me Love You" - Mario - 4 minutes 26 seconds.   Soulful, aching pleading for a much needed bit of loving.

"22,"- Night Beds 3 minutes 44 seconds   A journey into the mists of ethereal loving.

# The "Big O Orgasm"!

## What is a "Big O" Orgasm?

This very mysterious and very big OMG Orgasm is a wild and crazy sex obsessed ectoplasm type of protozoan critter residing in the human autonomic nervous system that chooses, at strategic moments in it's singularly focused lifestyle, to very loudly announce to anyone within hearing distance, that it is actually "coming" rather than "going. This is due to a sudden violently explosive discharge of accumulated sexual excitement and total loss of self control when "coming", or due to a turbulent buildup of aggravation, and sometimes aggression, accompanied by a total loss of tolerance and patience when "going".

The inclusion of a vocal high pitched "**OMG**" when "coming" is frequently employed to add emphasis and drama when the organism is finally approaching it's point of arrival.

The opposite statement, "I'm going" is usually accompanied by acronyms such as "**WTF**" delivered in gruff, dismissive, irritated and disappointed verbal tones together with copious spittle discharges and frequently accompanied by the sound of doors slamming hard and spirited middle finger presentations.

## How Do I Make My Orgasms Come or Go in the Direction I Desire?

If you you have sufficient privacy it is suggested that you sprinkle small directional signs in areas like the bedroom, kitchen, garage, broom closet, crawl space, garden shed, or anywhere where these loud exclamations seem to occur the most. They will at least offer a helpful guide to show where your orgasm should be coming from. Likewise, when it is going, an inconspicuous compass, a map or even a plane ticket to an exotic location hanging from a chain around the neck, can also be helpful when discerning a preferred direction of travel.

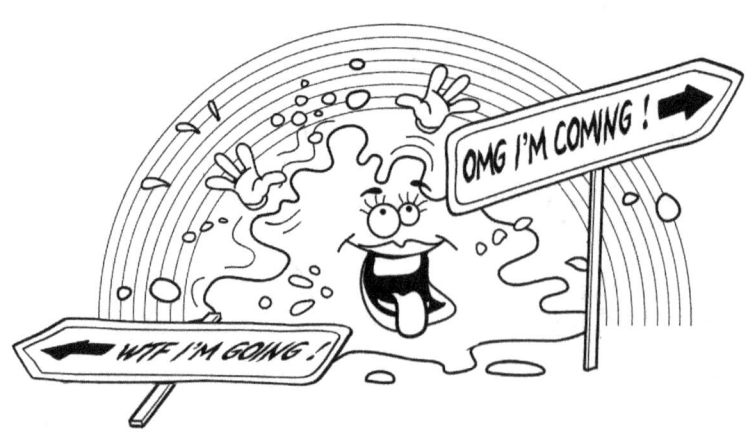

## Which God Works Best for the "OMG" Part ?

Most religions have a Deity that will almost certainly be trusted to be there at the end, "when you are going", and you can bet that they will be there on all the other occasions, "when you are coming". After establishing contact by calling out the "G" word a few times they somewhat predictably and dutifully jump in and do everything they can to actively augment the earth shattering experience that you, and hopefully your partner, if there is one, will remember and relish for all of the next few milliseconds. These beneficent Gods well know that their place in this particular orgasmic human activity will always be secure as long as they show up at exactly the right moment to show their support, their encouragement and the right path to heavenly bliss and rainbows either for all time or just this one very lust filled and passionate moment.

## How Many Times Can a Woman Climax at One Time ?

According to studies 7 in 10 women are able to climax numerous times with their partner (and some hit the big 'O' 20 times in a single session ! )
In fact, hitting the big 'O' more than once during a steamy session is common in most relationships, these studies show.
Two per cent of British women claim they are able to climax 20 times during their time "beneath" the sheets. There is no mention of how many climaxes they have "above" the sheets however.
For those of you that feel "left out" scientists claim to have found the ingredients for women to reach 'super-organisms'. Apparently these ingredients, which are a mix of yoga and bonding as well as relaxation, may enable a woman to climax as much as 100 times in one session.

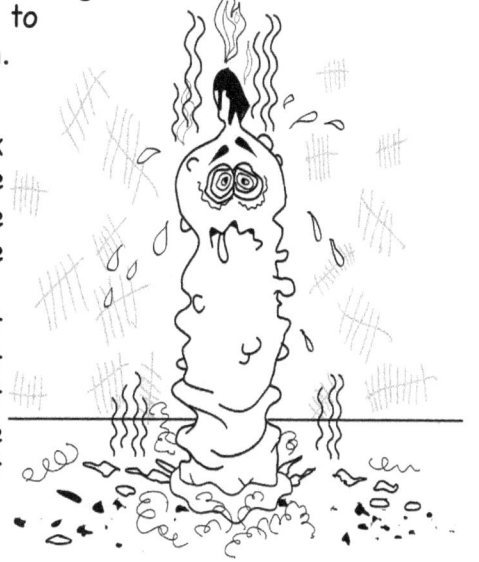

The study found that women who climax more than once during sex release more levels of oxytocin which is a love hormone that enables people to bond like Superglue with their lover.
This boosts immunity, induces a radiant glow and even protects against heart disease. There are even some doctors that think that experience these organisms are essential for overall wellbeing, if you don't spontaneously combust in the mean time.

# Blinded by The Night

Who would have ever thought that "vigorous sexual intercourse" could cause you to lose your eyesight. Well, it can and does happen, believe it or not.

The British Medical Journal recently reported that a 29 year old man arrived in hospital unable to see with one eye. He told doctors he had indulged in "vigorous sexual intercourse" all night !........So, what's with all that then ?

It turns out that really, really whopping orgasms can do your eyeballs harm. According to a paper this particular man presented himself to the emergency eye clinic and reported an obstruction in the central vision of his left eye, which he had noticed on waking that morning'.

The medics concluded his muscles were tense and he was holding his breath causing a blood vessel to pop in his eye.

Are there any other interesting problems, besides exploding eyeballs, that can be caused by explosive climaxes ? Well there are, according to an article by Men's Health there are 8 weird problems that can sometimes arise. Apart from the normal whole-body and pelvic sensation, flushing, increased heart rate, blood pressure, and heavy breathing as well as happiness, love and satisfaction there is also something called a peri-organism phenomena, physiological or psychological effects that fall beyond those usual responses. These can be...

**Hallucinations -** Flying sensation or even an out of body experiences.
**Sickness -** Sometimes called post-orgasm illness syndrome with flu like states of mind.
**Weakness -** This normally occurs with those who have sleep disorders.
**Crying -** This can be experienced as tearfulness, melancholy feelings, depression, anxiety, or agitation.
**Sneezing -** Starting with the activation of one part of the parasympathetic nervous system during orgasm that may actually trigger a different branch of it, sparking your sneezing symptoms.
**Pain -** Women can feel pain with an orgasm even if they don't experience pain with intercourse. Men with chronic prostate disease have also been known to experience pain with orgasm as well.
**Foot sensations -** A 2013 case report in the Journal of Sexual Medicine describes a 55-year-old woman complaining of "undesired orgasmic sensations" that originated in her left foot — which was the same feeling as when she was having sex with her husband.
**Headaches -** Orgasm induced headaches can range from several minutes to three hours, and may be alleviated with anti-migraine meds or pretreatment with propranolol.

# Color a Condom

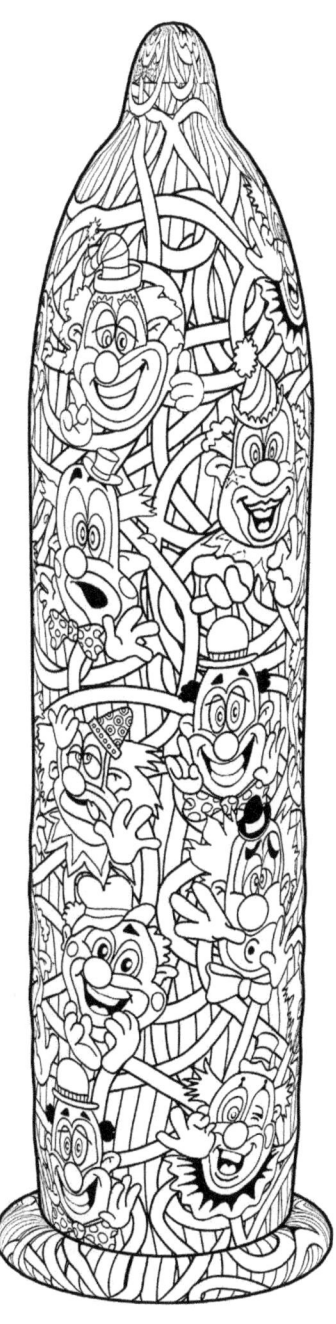

Before you succumb to any crying fits, cheer yourself up by coloring this sample 3D effect design from the companion book "The Cool Condom Coloring Book"! Get going with your coloring talents, this is one of the more tricky ones.

The **"Cool Condom Coloring Book,"** companion book, has 55 Johnny Jazzemup very varied and often challenging drawings to color!

# Sooty Sperm Discombobulations

Sad to say, it would appear that the size and shape of a man's sperm alters when exposed to diesel fumes. Recent research by The Chinese University is suggesting that sperm is adversely affected by sooty smoke. It is not known to what extent it affects fertility but researchers are concerned. Twenty six percent of men exposed to pollution were found to have the poorest sperm shape. Men living in high levels of pollution have more distorted sperm with a significant drop in normal size and shape.

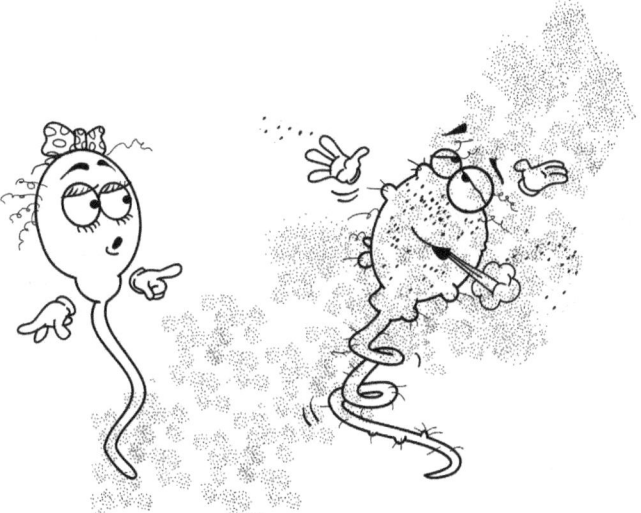

Experts analyzed exposure to sooty particles which are particularly linked to emissions of old diesel cars.

These particulates or particles - called PM2.5 - are so fine that they are breathed into the lungs and enter the blood stream potentially causing serious health problems. PM2.5 refers to atmospheric particulate matter (PM) that have a diameter of less than 2.5 micrometers. This is is about 3% the diameter of a human hair. These are even smaller than their counterparts PM10, which are particles that are 10 micrometres or less, and are also called fine particles.

Over the last few decades researchers have recorded a dramatic decline in the quantity and quality of sperm and IVF cycles (artificial fertilization of eggs) carried out in the UK show statistically that 49% are now linked to male fertility problems. Infertility is now a global public health concern.

There are dissenters such as Professor Allan Pacey, an expert in male fertility at the University of Sheffield who says that the jury is still out on the importance of sperm morphology which is not as important as people once thought and it's wise to be aware of it's limitation.

However Proffesor Pacey also says that "Air pollution probably does have the potential to negatively influence male reproductive health".

# Foreign Lingo for "Arriving at my Destination!"
## Or "Cumming" to be Precise...

People use both come and cum as a vulgar slang verb to mean the experience of having an orgasm, and/or ejaculating which means secreting semen from a male or any fluid that may be secreted from a female, at orgasm. A noun meaning semen or any fluid that may be secreted from a female during orgasm. Cum is the thick white fluid containing spermatozoa that is ejaculated by a male.

How does one say one is about to climax in other languages? The handy translations included here may, or may not be, entirely accurate but, they might offer some type of clue as to where in the proceedings your foreign partner may be heading. Judging on the many languages that use "cumming" it must be the most popular word in common usage worldwide.

Ever think about "going" to "Cumming"? It actually exists in Georgia US. Take your wellies if you ever go there and keep your orgasmic vocalizations to a minimum to avoid scaring those that have to live with the "Cumming" stuff all the time.

**Welsh**
Rydym yn cummi

**Polish**
CIEKAĆ

**German**
Ich bin cumming

**Japanese**
私はカミングしている

**Mongolian**
Би цангаж байна

**Hungarian**
jövök

**Croatian**
Ja sam cumming

**French**
Je suis cumming

**Swedish**
Jag kommer

**Uzbek**
Jeg er cumming

**Danish**
Jeg kommer

**Turkish**
Ben cumming

**Portugese**
Estou cumming

**Bosnian**
Ja sam cumming

**Russian**
я кончаю

**Czech**
Já jsem cumming

**Scots Gaelic**
Tha mi a 'cluinntinn

**Greek**
είμαι cumming

**Icelandic**
ég er cumming

**Dutch**
Ik cumming

**Slovac**
Ja som cumming

**Luxembourgish**
Ech sinn cumming

**Lithuanian**
aš cummingas

**Italian**
Sto cumming

**Estonian**
Ma cumming

**Australian**
What the hell was that?

**Indonesian**
saya cumming

**Latvian**
Es esmu cumming

**Nepali**
म कम गर्दै छु

**Samoan**
ua ou togi

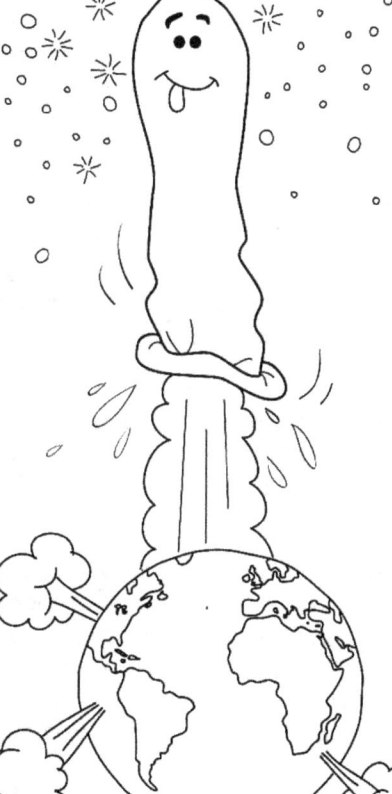

**Georgian**
მე კუმინგში ვარ

**Malay**
saya bersemangat

**Chichewa**
ndikuwongolera

**Xhosa**
I Ndiza cumming

**Romanian**
Sunt cumming

**Korean**
메신저

**Maori**
Ahau te cumming

**Punjabi**
ਮੈਂ ਕਮਿੰਗ ਕਰ ਰਿਹਾ ਹਾਂ

**Tajik**
ман келин хастам

**Norwegian**
Jeg er cumming

**Finish**
Olen cumming

**Basque**
zirikatzen ari naiz

**Zulu**
ngiyaqhubek

**Filipino**
Ja сам цумминг

**Shona**
ndiri kumira

**Yiddish**
איך בין קאמינג

**Irish**
Tá mé cumming

**Kyrgyz**
мен Камминг жатам

**Hindi**
मैं कमिंग रहा

**Serbian**
Ja сам цумминг

**Slovenian**
Sem cumming

**Macedonian**
Јас сум каминг

**Romanian**
Sunt cumming

**Zulu**
Ngiyaqhubeka

**Spanish**
Estoy cumming

**Bulgarian**
Аз съм cumming

**Lao**
ຂ້ອຍພະເຈົ້າໄດ້ cummin

**Albanian**
Unë jam cumming

**Yaroba**
Mo n cumming

**Swahili**
Mimi ni cumming

**Azerbaijani**
Mən cumming edirəm

**Igbo**
Ana m arụ ọrụ

**Chinese**
"我正在康复"

# 15 Favorite Places to Make Out

**A BED**
For 90 % of the time a good old dependable bed works perfectly. You know how to quickly navigate all the misshapen lumps and squeaky springs and there is no subsequent traveling issue apart from a quick trip to bathroom to brush your teeth and have a leak.

**THE BACK SEAT**
Ah, the old back seat trick, commonly used when the car is too small to use the front seat and the gear stick takes over too much of the action when the feet are caught sticking out of the windows wrapped around the rear view mirror. Always a favorite lay-by pastime when the long road behind, and ahead, get visually boring and you need more than just a simple potty break. The windows usually get all steamed up pretty quickly so no worries about a growing crowd watching the action.

**THE COUCH**
When you realize that the movie you are about to view for the evening was the same one that the two of you have already watched for three nights previously and washing the dishes piled up in the sink is not an option then the couch is the best place to embark on a few hours of labored lust and six-pack fueled passion.

**AN ELEVATOR**
A great idea when a little spice is needed to attain new heights of hedonistic titillation between floor levels. The best tip is to start in the basement and immediately shoot off to the top floor. Not recommended when the elevator is located in the local police station however.

**THE OCEAN**
Every thunderous wave that smashes against your writhing bodies presents a powerful and explosive thrusting assist, each crashing wave making penetration deeper and deeper. Poisonous jellyfish brushing gently against goose pimpled butts together with the twitching fins of circling sharks give this fun location a sense of adventurous intensity and urgency that other less intimidating locations might lack.

**UNDER A WATERFALL**
This is always a romantic location on a hot summers day. Embracing under a cool playful cascade of sun soaked water droplets will melt any heart and invoke a sense of passion that only a large group of extreme kayakers shooting the falls could possibly interrupt.

**MOVIE THEATRE**
If the advertisements are longer than the movie a great way to pass the time is to make out under protective extra large buckets of popcorn. Make sure you are in a back seat and not in front of or not right under the movie projector, as having silhouettes of couples bouncing up and down right there on the movie screen can be downright distracting. Recently a couple in a San Antonio cinema were spotted romping by a 'shocked' worker in a theatre at around midnight, according to the police report. The pair were both jailed and charged with public lewdness. They were reported to be having sex really fast but obviously not quite fast enough to avoid being caught in flagrante delicto.

## A SWIMMING POOL
Certainly not in a public swimming pool as that would be unhygienic, but if you own a pool then this certainly is a great way to break into a few new swimming strokes. Carefully try out on a diving board and when you both reach that magical moment, bounce of it into the water while interlocked. Amazingly trippy.

## IN A LIBRARY
Reading such publications as Lady Chatterly's Lover in a library will set the stage for lust filled indulgences when the library closes. Get that ladder ready, the hair up and the specs out as if you know exactly what ISBN numbers turn you on the most.

## SWINGING IN A HAMMOCK
First, before doing anything else, make sure that the tree on both sides of the hammock is not about to fall over with the most rigorous shake. Then determine if there are any squirrels in the area that are on the lookout for nuts. If all is clear, swing that hammock around every which way until those Summer leaves fall like Autumn has arrived early.

## THE MILE HIGH CLUB
The advise from flight attendants is basically don't do it in public, do it quietly and don't act suspicious during entire flight. Also no cheating, you have to wait patiently until the plane really is a mile high. Doing the dirty deed while the aircraft is still on the taxiway is considered "too previous". As a suggestion it is also a good idea to have an appropriate speech prepared when you leave the toilets and find all the passengers clapping, whooping and hollering.

## ON A SKI LIFT
Before you indulge your lust, first make sure that you are safely and firmly attached to your seat and there is only soft powdery snow beneath you, no exposed rocks or tree stumps visible. Next check out your partner for any signs of frostbite or sunburn. You don't want to make it worse. Make sure both your skis are pointing in the direction you want them and are not entangled in any way. After that secure your hats and gloves so they don't fall off when you get going. Check to see if there are lift posts in the way or if the ski patrol is nearby. If all looks good get going pretty quickly in case you fall right off the end of the ride while right in the middle of the ride.

## UNDER THE STARS
Just about anywhere under the stars is magical as they add a perfect backdrop to those otherworldly transitory feelings of far out beatitude and exultation that only the very heavens themselves are able to conjure up.

# The Ups, Downs, Ins and Outs of.........

We all know what the "upside "is so let's go straight to the "downside" for a bit of contrast. Jacking/jerking off, as we were all told when we were kids, can eventually make you go blind or even grow hairs in the palms of your hand ! This is no longer just a myth that has been disproven many times but is also something that occurs naturally after years of hard work and endless effort, with or without a condom. Eventually the hairs grow on your palm and the blindness reveals itself when one's ability to read and see printed type clearly begins to fail. Quite suddenly, while reading a book, the printed word starts to fade in front of one's very eyes and one has to squint in order to read it. This is usually a strong indication that through the years one has unfortunately gone a little bit overboard with the regularly scheduled unabated practice sessions.

If this curious phenomenon ever happens to you just lay off the "diddling" for a few years and your eyesight and the visibility of book print will return to normal once again. Unfortunately though the curly hairs on your palms will remain stubbornly visible for everyone to see when you open your hand for change at the grocery counter.

## Galloping the Maggot
### DUDES

| | |
|---|---|
| JAPO (Jack Off Pass Out ) | Churning Butter |
| Applying the Hand Brake | Chucking Custard |
| Badgering the Witness | Pumping the Stump |
| Playing the Skin Flute | Rubbing One Out |
| Jackin' the Beanstalk | Croaking the Frog |
| Beef Stroganoff | Making Jam |
| Spreading Jelly | Wanking |
| Tossing Off | Gurning at God |
| Disseminating | Killing the Kids |
| Making Chowder | Tossing the Salad |
| Milking the Lizard | Reaming the Demon |
| Cleaning your Rifle | Playing the Skin Flute |
| Stirring the Batter | Jacking it in San Diego |
| Painting the Ceiling | Giving a Dirty Handshake |
| Choking the Cyclops | Dancing around the Mapole |
| Dishonorable Discharge | Warming the Alter Boy's Dinner |

Want to clear a snotty nose ? Apparently masturbation clears congestion as well. During an orgasm the muscles contract around the body, including inside the nose, which can temporarily relieve sinus pressure for both men and women. The hanky you carry around with you to wipe your nose is now freed up by other more vigorous and pleasurable pursuits.

# Stuffing the Envelope
## DUDETTES

Taking a Self-Guided Tuna Boat Tour
Having a Night in with The Girls
Auditioning the Finger Puppets
Tiptoeing Through the Two Lips
Buttering the Whisker Biscuit
Roughing up the Suspect
Unbuttoning the Fur Coat
Opening the Ham Wallet
Polishing the Pearl
Circling the Wagon
Clubbing the Clam
Airing the Orchid
Rolling the Dough
Singing Soprano
Impeaching Bush
Menage a Mois
Tracing Eights
Finger Painting
Muffin Buffin'
Pearl Fishing
Finding Nemo
Juicing
Tiggling
Shebopping
Low-Fiving
Jilling Off
Elabiorating
Making Soup
Fingerbating
Bliss-Torizing
Brainstorming
Procrasturbating
Pleasure Cruising

Hitting the Self Destruct Button
Making a Fish Finger Sandwich
Streaming the Goo Goo Dolls
Getting lost in the Deep End
Making a Flesh Smoothie
Undressing the Wound
Dancing in the Dark
Slip-A-Dee Doo-Dah
Guided Meditation
Plunging the Clunge
Embracing Feminism
Raiding the Fridge
Tripping the Switch
Micro Massaging
Diddling the Kids
Saucing the Taco
Wet and Wilding
Gilding the Lily
Battery Testing
Womansplaining
Pussitioning
TriggeringZ
Launching
Ecstasizing
Diddle a Skittle
Taming the Shrew
Soaking the Sponge
Checking Your Pulse
Pushing Your Button
Singing in the Shower
Beating around the Bush
Visiting the Finger Vault
Double Clicking the Mouse

81

# Safe Sex is GOOD for You!

## It is estimated that 183,009 people have sex every hour.

### Boosts Brain Power
Coventry University researchers discovered that those who engaged regular sexual activity scored higher on tests that measured verbal fluency and ability to visually perceive objects and the spaces between them.

### Reduces Anxiety
People who reported more sexual intercourse had lower blood pressure when performing stressful tasks.

### Heart Health
A study at Queens University in Belfast found that having sex three times a week could actually halve the risk of heart attack or stroke.

### Makes You Happy
One study estimated that boosting intercourse from once a month to once a week was the happiness equivalent of getting a $50,000 raise and a free extra jam doughnut with a cup of joe at the local coffee joint.

### Boosts Your Immunity
New Scientist Magazine reports that researchers speculate that moderate sexual activity exposes you to other people's bugs, boosting the immune system.

### Soothes Your Pain
Orgasms don't just feel good; they ease pain.

### Decreases Neuroticism
Neuroticism tends to make people unhappy, but sex wipes worries away, making neurotic newlyweds as satisfied as their relaxed counterparts.

### Reduces Prostate Cancer Risk
Men who ejaculated the most – 21 times a month or more – were about one-third less likely to develop prostate cancer than those who ejaculated between four and seven times a month. The jury is still out on when and if adding extra ejaculation to your life is helpful, Research on the topic has been somewhat contradictory however.

### Health Benefits of Condoms
They can actually boost vaginal health. Apart from the obvious which is preventing sexually transmitted diseases — condoms can potentially improve vaginal health by increasing levels of "friendly" bacteria and preventing minor infections.

### Sex Rarely Causes Cardiac Arrest
According to the American Heart Association sex rarely causes cardiac arrest even in cardiac patients. In a research letter in the Journal of the American College of Cardiology study by Dr. Aapo Aro (Cedars-Sinai Heart Institute, Los Angeles, CA) was found to be "reassuring."

# ...but Unsafe Sex is NOT!

**Silliness aside folks, these few pages should be taken very seriously so PLEASE PAY ATTENTION TO THE FOLLOWING PAGES!**

Consistent condom use provides substantial protection against the acquisition of many STDs, including statistically significant reduction of risk against HIV, chlamydia, gonorrhea, herpes, and syphilis.

## STD/STIs

- Chlamydia
- Gonorrhea
- Genital Herpes
- HIV/AIDS
- Human Papillomavirus (HPV)
- Molluscum Contagiosum
- Scabies
- Yeast in Men
- Chancroid
- Syphilis
- Bacterial Vaginosis
- Trichomoniasis
- Viral Hepatitis
- Hepatitis B and C
- HPV Warts
- Vaginal Yeast
- Vaginosis
- Pelvic Inflammatory Disease

Total U.S. cases of chlamydia, gonorrhea and syphilis are higher than ever. Syphilis cases alone climbed 19 percent between 2014 and 2015, according to new data released this week by the Centers for Disease Control and Prevention.

There are more than 1.5 million cases of chlamydia nationwide, as well as 400,000 cases of gonorrhea and almost 24,000 cases of the most infectious stages of syphilis, according to the new data. Teens and young adults ages 15 to 24 account for nearly two-thirds of diagnosed cases of chlamydia and half of gonorrhea cases.

STDs cost the U.S. health care system nearly $16 billion a year, according to the CDC. And chlamydia, gonorrhea and syphilis are curable with antibiotics, but most STD cases go undiagnosed and untreated. That puts those infected at greater risk for serious health threats, including infertility, chronic pain and HIV infection.

STD rates are rising, and many of the country's systems for preventing STDs have eroded. If expanded services are not mobilized or rebuilt the human and economic burden will continue to grow.

# STD/STI Statistics

According to a new CDC report in 2016 sex diseases in the US surge to record high with more than 2 MILLION cases of chlamydia, gonorrhea and syphilis.

**Most new cases - 1.6m in 2016 - involved chlamydia.**

**Gonorrhea increased mostly among men, up 22 percent in a year.**

**Syphilis cases rocketed up 18 percent to 28,000 nationally.**

- More than half of all people will have an STD/STI at some point in their lifetime.[1]
- Recent estimates from the Centers for Disease Control and Infection show that there are 19.7 million new STIs every year in the U.S.
- The total estimated direct cost of STIs annually in the U.S. is $15.6 billion (2010 US dollars).
- Each year, one in four teens contracts an STD/STI.
- One in two sexually active persons will contract an STD/STI by age 25.
- It is estimated that as many as one in five Americans have genital herpes, a lifelong (but manageable) infection, yet up to 90 percent of those with herpes
- Some estimates suggest that by 2025 up to 40% of all men and half of all women could be infected with genital herpes.
- Each year, there are almost 3 million new cases of chlamydia, many of which are in adolescents and young adults.
- More than 42 percent of Americans between the ages of 18 and 59 are infected with genital human papillomavirus.
- At least 15 percent of all American women who are infertile can attribute it to tubal damage caused by pelvic inflammatory disease (PID), the result of an untreated STD. Consistent condom use reduces the risk of recurrent PID and related complications: significantly, women who reported regular use of condoms in one study were 60 percent less likely to become infertile.

Apparently a big societal problem to overcome is the embarrassment of having an STD. Unfortunately they carry enormous stigma in the US which makes it hard for people to come forward for treatment. So, overcome the embarrassment factor, do yourself a favor and get tested regularly.

## Centers for Disease Control and Prevention Report 2017

In 2016, Americans were infected with more than 2 million new cases of gonorrhea, syphilis and chlamydia, the highest number of these sexually transmitted diseases ever reported.

The agency's annual Sexually Transmitted Disease Surveillance Report shows that more than 1.6 million of the new cases were from chlamydia, 470,000 were from gonorrhea and nearly 28,000 cases were of primary and secondary syphilis. Secondary syphilis is the most contagious form of the disease, according to the CDC. While all of these can be cured by antibiotics, many people go undiagnosed and untreated.

Only those three STDs are required by law to be reported to the CDC by physicians. When you include HIV, herpes and more of the dozens of diseases which can be transmitted sexually but which are not tracked, the CDC estimates there are more than 20 million new cases of STDs in the United States each year. At least half occur in young people ages 15 to 24.

The most common STD is chlamydia. It's caused by the bacteria chlamydia trachomatis, and like most STDs, is easily transmitted by all forms of sexual activity -- oral, vaginal or anal -- as well as during childbirth. Chlamydia is known as a "silent" infection, because most people have no symptoms, which means it often goes untreated. In women, it can ultimately cause pelvic inflammatory disease that can scar and affect fertility. In men, it can cause testicular pain and swelling.

Gonorrhea is another bacterial STD that can be silent, but often displays symptoms such as burning during urination and vaginal or penile discharge. If caught anally, it can create itching, bleeding and painful bowel movements. If not treated, gonorrhea can cause severe and permanent health problems, including long-term pain and infertility.

Syphilis is the most serious bacterial STD. Left untreated, syphilis can affect the brain, heart and other organs of the body, ultimately leading to death. It's called the "Great Pretender," because the symptoms of syphilis which include rashes and chancres, or sores, fever, swollen lymph glands, sore throat, headaches, muscles aches and fatigue, mimic other diseases. As the disease progresses, the symptoms go away, and progress silently to it's most deadly stage.

# STD/STI Statistics

According to a new CDC report in 2016 sex diseases in the US surge to record high with more than 2 MILLION cases of chlamydia, gonorrhea and syphilis.

Most new cases - 1.6m in 2016 - involved chlamydia.

Gonorrhea increased mostly among men, up 22 percent in a year.

Syphilis cases rocketed up 18 percent to 28,000 nationally.

- More than half of all people will have an STD/STI at some point in their lifetime.[1]
- Recent estimates from the Centers for Disease Control and Infection show that there are 19.7 million new STIs every year in the U.S.
- The total estimated direct cost of STIs annually in the U.S. is $15.6 billion (2010 US dollars).
- Each year, one in four teens contracts an STD/STI.
- One in two sexually active persons will contract an STD/STI by age 25.
- It is estimated that as many as one in five Americans have genital herpes, a lifelong (but manageable) infection, yet up to 90 percent of those with herpes are unaware they have it.
- Some estimates suggest that by 2025 up to 40% of all men and half of all women could be infected with genital herpes.
- Each year, there are almost 3 million new cases of chlamydia, many of which are in adolescents and young adults.
- More than 42 percent of Americans between the ages of 18 and 59 are infected with genital human papillomavirus.
- At least 15 percent of all American women who are infertile can attribute it to tubal damage caused by pelvic inflammatory disease (PID), the result of an untreated STD. Consistent condom use reduces the risk of recurrent PID and related complications: significantly, women who reported regular use of condoms in one study were 60 percent less likely to become infertile.

Apparently a big societal problem to overcome is the embarrassment of having an STD. Unfortunately they carry enormous stigma in the US which makes it hard for people to come forward for treatment. So, overcome the embarrassment factor, do yourself a favor and get tested regularly.

## Centers for Disease Control and Prevention Report 2017

In 2016, Americans were infected with more than 2 million new cases of gonorrhea, syphilis and chlamydia, the highest number of these sexually transmitted diseases ever reported.

The agency's annual Sexually Transmitted Disease Surveillance Report shows that more than 1.6 million of the new cases were from chlamydia, 470,000 were from gonorrhea and nearly 28,000 cases were of primary and secondary syphilis. Secondary syphilis is the most contagious form of the disease, according to the CDC. While all of these can be cured by antibiotics, many people go undiagnosed and untreated.

Only those three STDs are required by law to be reported to the CDC by physicians. When you include HIV, herpes and more of the dozens of diseases which can be transmitted sexually but which are not tracked, the CDC estimates there are more than 20 million new cases of STDs in the United States each year. At least half occur in young people ages 15 to 24.

The most common STD is chlamydia. It's caused by the bacteria chlamydia trachomatis, and like most STDs, is easily transmitted by all forms of sexual activity -- oral, vaginal or anal -- as well as during childbirth. Chlamydia is known as a "silent" infection, because most people have no symptoms, which means it often goes untreated. In women, it can ultimately cause pelvic inflammatory disease that can scar and affect fertility. In men, it can cause testicular pain and swelling.

Gonorrhea is another bacterial STD that can be silent, but often displays symptoms such as burning during urination and vaginal or penile discharge. If caught anally, it can create itching, bleeding and painful bowel movements. If not treated, gonorrhea can cause severe and permanent health problems, including long-term pain and infertility.

Syphilis is the most serious bacterial STD. Left untreated, syphilis can affect the brain, heart and other organs of the body, ultimately leading to death. It's called the "Great Pretender," because the symptoms of syphilis which include rashes and chancres, or sores, fever, swollen lymph glands, sore throat, headaches, muscles aches and fatigue, mimic other diseases. As the disease progresses, the symptoms go away, and progress silently to it's most deadly stage.

# Chlamydia

Chlamydia is a sexually-transmitted disease that can infect males and females.

It stems from bacteria called chlamydia trachomatis. It is passed through contact, via vaginal, anal or oral sex.

If left untreated it can damage a woman's fallopian tubes and cause infertility. In very rare cases it can cause infertility in men too.

## What are the symptoms ?

The majority of people do not feel symptoms of chlamydia. Doctors recommend getting regular STD tests (urine test or swab) to detect it.

However, some do experience some side effects.

Symptoms in women:

Abnormal vaginal discharge

Burning feeling when you urinate

Pain in the eyes

Pain in the abdomen

Pain in the pelvis

Pain during sex

Vaginal bleeding

Symptoms in men:

Discharge from the penis

Burning feeling when you urinate

Rarely: Pain and swelling in one or both testicles

Symptoms of chlamydia after anal sex:

Pain in the rectum

Discharge

Bleeding

## How is it treated ?

The infection is easily treated with antibiotics.

Doctors typically prescribe oral antibiotics, usually azithromycin (Zithromax) or doxycycline.

# Syphilis

A chronic bacterial disease, syphilis can be contracted by other means but is typically a sexually-transmitted disease.

In very rare cases, it can be spread through prolonged kissing, as well as the more common routes of transmission: vaginal, anal and oral sex.

It comes from the bacteria Treponema pallidum.

## What are the symptoms ?

Sufferers develop sores, though these can often go ignored.

The infection develops in stages.

## Stage one:

Small, painless sores (like ulcers) on genitals or in the mouth.

Appear within 10-90 days after exposure.

They disappear within six weeks, and do not leave a scar, before developing to stage two.

## Stage two:

Rosy rash on the palms of the hand and soles of the feet

Moist warts in the groin.

White patches inside the mouth and swollen glands

Fever

Weight loss

This all fades away without treatment before developing into stage three

Latent syphilis:

Dormant, no symptoms

## Stage three:

Without treatment it can progress to more severe issues with the heart, brain and nerves causing...

| | |
|---|---|
| Paralysis | Deafness |
| Blindness | Impotence |
| Dementia | Death |

## How is it treated ?

In the early stages, patients can receive an injection of Benzathine penicillin G. This will not undo the internal damage but will eliminate the infection.

For those with latent syphilis - and are unsure how long they had it - doctors recommend having three doses of the penicillin injection, seven days apart from each other.

# Gonorrhea

A very similar STD to chlamydia, gonorrhea is also bacterial, spread through contact. It stems from bacteria called neisseria gonorrhoeae.

## What are the symptoms?

Women typically do not see symptoms; men do.

When a woman does experience symptoms, they are very mild and easily mistaken for a bladder infection.

Doctors recommend getting regular STD tests (urine test or swab) to detect it.

Symptoms in men:

Burning feeling when you urinate

A white, yellow, or green discharge from the penis

Rarely: Painful or swollen testicles

Symptoms in women:

Burning feeling when you urinate

Increased vaginal discharge

Vaginal bleeding between periods

## How is it treated ?

Gonorrhea is curable with antibiotics, though health officials fear this may be the first 'untreatable' STD as the bacteria builds up resistance to our standard methods of treatment.

The CDC recommends treating the infection with a combination of two antibiotics: azithromycin and ceftriaxone.

The infection has already become immune to penicillin, tetracycline and fluoroquinolones.

Increasingly, gonorrhea is building up a resistance to the individual drugs.

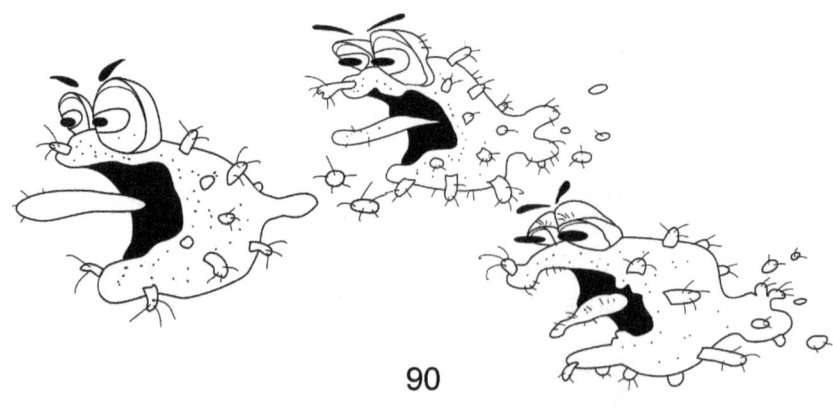

# Beware of the Gonorrhea Superbug!

Gonorrhea, commonly known as "the clap" or "the drip," is one of the most common sexually transmitted diseases there is. Anyone who is sexually active is at risk and any kind of sex, including anal and oral sex, can pass it along.

Lately a new untreatable strain of gonorrhea has been discovered. This super bug, formally named H041, an untreatable strain, is rapidly spreading across the world putting millions of lives at risk. No known form of antibiotic can treat it. It is largely caused by oral sex and a decline in condom use.

The sexually transmitted bacteria can live at the back of the throat and, because of this, they have evolved immunity to antibiotics used to treat common throat infections. Experts from the WHO have said it is 'only a matter of time' before last-resort gonorrhea antibiotics would be of no use at all. Resistance to last-case antibiotics has already been reported in 50 countries. Only three potential new gonorrhea drugs are in development and there is no guarantee any will prove effective in final-stage trials.

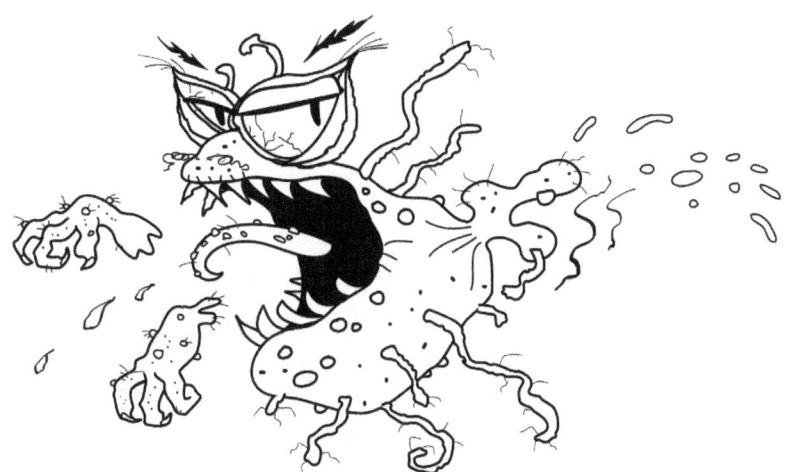

Men and women with gonorrhea often don't show symptoms and may not experience anything at all, others will see symptoms between one and 14 days after they've been infected. The infection can be contracted and passed through oral, vaginal and anal sex so it's important for partners to get tested regularly. Untreated gonorrhea can cause a multitude of problems but abstinence and condoms are the best ways to prevent it.

According to the CDC, there are 700,000 new cases of gonorrhea in the U.S each year and 340 million new cases globally. There are several reasons it's spreading. Decreasing condom use, increased urbanization and travel, poor infection detection rates, and inadequate or failed treatment all contribute to this increase.

# HIV/AIDS

HIV stands for human immunodeficiency virus. It weakens a person's immune system by destroying important cells that fight disease and infection. No effective cure exists for HIV. But with proper medical care, HIV can be controlled.

HIV is a virus spread through certain body fluids that attacks the body's immune system, specifically the CD4 cells, often called T cells. Over time, HIV can destroy so many of these cells that the body can't fight off infections and disease. These special cells help the immune system fight off infections. Untreated, HIV reduces the number of CD4 cells (T cells) in the body. This damage to the immune system makes it harder and harder for the body to fight off infections and some other diseases. Opportunistic infections or cancers take advantage of a very weak immune system and signal that the person has AIDS.

No effective cure currently exists, but with proper medical care, HIV can be controlled. The medicine used to treat HIV is called antiretroviral therapy or ART. If taken the right way, every day, this medicine can dramatically prolong the lives of many people infected with HIV, keep them healthy, and greatly lower their chance of infecting others. Before the introduction of ART in the mid-1990s, people with HIV could progress to AIDS in just a few years. Today, someone diagnosed with HIV and treated before the disease is far advanced can live nearly as long as someone who does not have HIV.

There are three stages:

**Stage 1:** Acute HIV infection

**Stage 2:** Clinical latency (HIV inactivity or dormancy)

**Stage 3:** Acquired immunodeficiency syndrome (AIDS)

Stage 3 is the most severe phase of HIV infection. People with AIDS have such badly damaged immune systems that they get an increasing number of severe illnesses, called opportunistic illnesses.

Without treatment, people with AIDS typically survive about 3 years. Common symptoms of AIDS include chills, fever, sweats, swollen lymph glands, weakness, and weight loss. People are diagnosed with AIDS when their CD4 cell count drops below 200 cells/mm or if they develop certain opportunistic illnesses. People with AIDS can have a high viral load and be very infectious.

To find places near you that offer confidential HIV testing,
Visit gettested.cdc.gov,

Text your ZIP code to KNOW IT (566948), or

Call 1-800-CDC-INFO (1-800-232-4636).

You can also use a home testing kit, available for purchase in most pharmacies and online.

After you get tested, it's important to find out the result of your test so you can talk to your health care provider about treatment options if you're HIV-positive or learn ways to prevent getting HIV if you're HIV-negative.

# HIV in the US

In 2014, there were an estimated 37,600 new HIV infections—down from 45,700 in 2008.

In 2016, 39,782 people received an HIV diagnosis. The annual number of new diagnoses declined by 5% from 2011 to 2015.

If we look at HIV infections* by transmission category, we see that gay, bisexual, and other men who have sex with men are most at risk. In 2014, gay and bisexual men accounted for 70% of all new HIV infections. In the same year, individuals infected through heterosexual sex made up 23% of all new HIV infections. (This does not include black/African Americans who are Hispanic.)

HIV diagnoses by race and ethnicity, show that African Americans are most affected by HIV. In 2016, African Americans made up only 12% of the US population but had 44% of all new HIV diagnoses. Additionally, Hispanic/Latinos are also strongly affected. They made up 18% of the US population but had 25% of all new HIV diagnoses.(Hispanics/Latinos can be of any race.)

Young people aged 13-24 are especially affected by HIV. In 2015, they comprised 16% of the US population but accounted for 22% of all new HIV diagnoses. All young people are not equally at risk, however. Young gay and bisexual men accounted for 84% of all new HIV diagnoses in people aged 13-24 in 2015, and young, African American gay and bisexual men are even more severely affected.

## Do people still die from HIV ?

Yes. In the United States, 6,721 people died from HIV and AIDS in 2014. HIV remains a significant cause of death for certain populations. In 2014, it was the 8th leading cause of death for those aged 25-34 and 9th for those aged 35-44.

## Do some parts of the country have more HIV than other parts ?

Yes. HIV is largely an urban disease, with most cases occurring in metropolitan areas with 500,000 or more people. The South has the highest number of people living with HIV, but if population size is taken into account, the Northeast has the highest rate of people living with HIV. (Rates are the number of cases of disease per 100,000 people. Rates allow comparisons between groups of different sizes.)

HIV disease continues to be a serious health issue for parts of the world. Worldwide, there were about 1.8 million new cases of HIV in 2016. About 36.7 million people were living with HIV around the world in 2016, and 19.5 million of them were receiving medicines to treat HIV, called antiretroviral therapy (ART). An estimated 1 million people died from AIDS-related illnesses in 2016. Sub-Saharan Africa, which bears the heaviest burden of HIV and AIDS worldwide, accounts for about 64% of all new HIV infections. Other regions significantly affected by HIV and AIDS include Asia and the Pacific, Latin America and the Caribbean, and Eastern Europe and Central Asia.

The above information has been condensed from the CDC web pages. For more information see CDCs Global AIDS website www.cdc.gov to see what CDC is doing in the global fight against HIV.

# HIV and Sex Education

The status of sexual health education varies substantially throughout the USA and is insufficient in many areas.

In most states, fewer than half of high schools teach all 16 critical topics that CDC recommends for effective sex education. Specifically, many schools do not include prevention information that relates to the needs of young men who have sex with men. Many also argue that sex education is not starting early enough. A 2014 CDC study found half or less than half of the middle schools in every state teaching all 16 topics.

Sex education has also been declining over time across the country. The percentage of US schools in which students are required to receive instruction on HIV prevention decreased from 64% in 2000 to 41% in 2014.

www.avert.org  Global Information and Education on HIV and AIDS

---

### The US National HIV/AIDS Strategy's Mission Statement

"The United States will become a place where new HIV infections are rare, and when they do occur, every person, regardless of age, gender, race/ethnicity, sexual orientation, gender identity, or socio-economic circumstance, will have unfettered access to high quality, life-extending care, free from stigma and discrimination."

---

## Aids Organizations

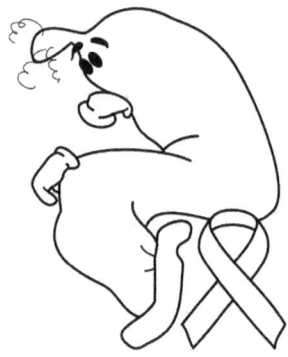

1. The Global Fund
2. Center for AIDS Research, UC San Diego
3. UNAIDS
4. The Elton John AIDS Foundation
5. Treatment Action Campaign
6. The Rush Foundation
7. AmfAR
8. Avert
9. https://en.wikipedia.org/wiki/Category:HIV/AIDS_organizations
https://en.wikipedia.org/wiki/Category:HIV/AIDS_prevention_organizations

# Not Forgetting Our Environment

Flushing condoms down the toilet is **NOT RECOMMENDED**. Condoms can clog your plumbing, clog your sewers or even end up in the water supply. If condoms are disposed of via the toilet, they are usually fished out early on in the water-recycling process and transported to a landfill. However, if not caught early, condoms can remain with other water waste and may be sent out into sea where fish or birds may try to eat them.

Latex is biodegradable (when not under water). It is an all-natural substance made from the sap of rubber trees. Latex condoms are not composed of 100 percent latex, though. Another material used to make condoms, lambskin, is also biodegradable, but it does not protect against sexually transmitted infections (STIs) and HIV. Condoms made of polyurethane, a plastic material, do not break down at all. They cannot be recycled so don't throw them in the recycling bin!

Remember, that apart from just condoms. all plastic items are a threat to our environment as well. Try to use plastic bags more than once and try to use eco friendly reusable and recycled shopping bags. Plastics frequently pollute waterways, public areas and are even washing into our increasingly polluted oceans.

We humans, and all ocean life will thank you for being caring and responsible !

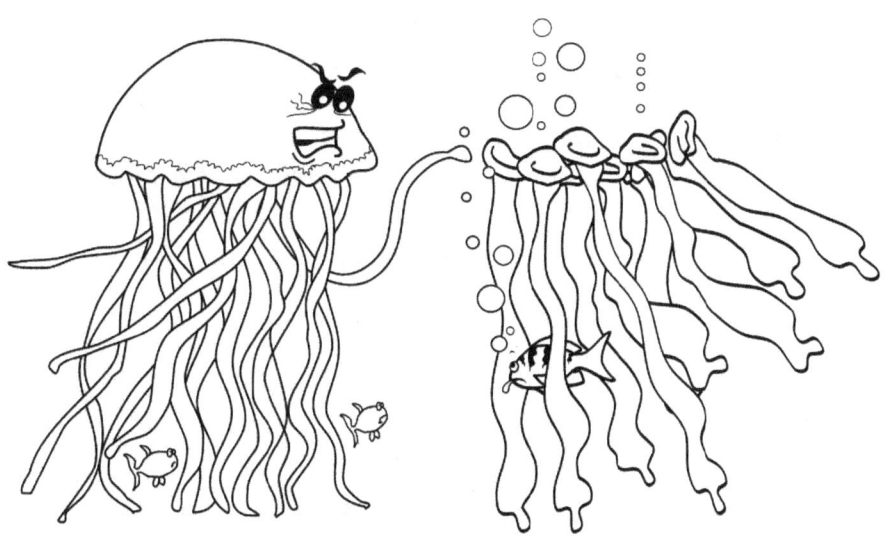

# Warnings

### Know Your Rights
Insist on using a condom, refuse sex without a condom and use a new condom over shared sex toys.

### You cannot reuse condoms.
It is surprising just how many sexually active people believe this to be true, but condoms are meant to be used just once only and then discarded in an environmentally responsible way afterwards.

### Lubricants
Latex condoms can be damaged by oil-based lubricants.

### Smoking
Because it reduces blood flow to the penis, smoking can shorten the average penis by up to 0.4 inches (1 cm) studies have found.

### Smuggling
Condoms have also been used to smuggle alcohol, cocaine, heroin, and other drugs across borders and into prisons by filling the condom with drugs, tying it in a knot and then either swallowing it or inserting it into the rectum. Warning, these methods are very dangerous and potentially lethal. If the condom breaks, the drugs inside become absorbed into the bloodstream and body and can cause an overdose likely resulting in death.

**Remember, it's ALWAYS better to be safe than sorry !**

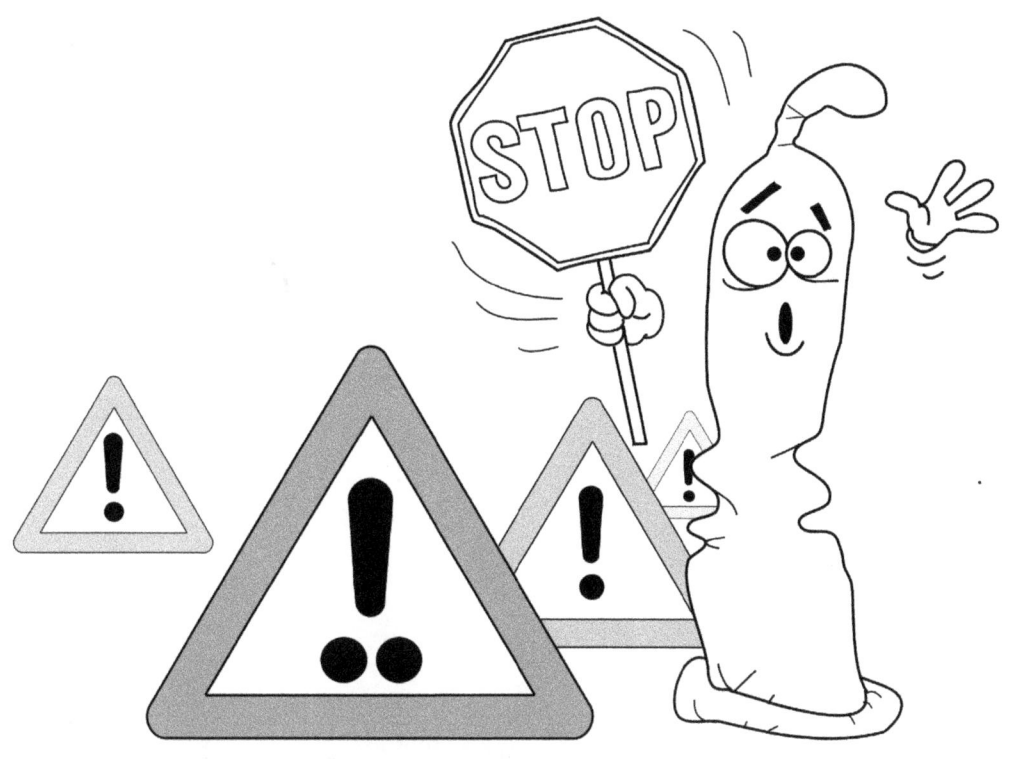

# The Cool Condom
## Coloring Book

Don't forget to check out the companion book "The Cool Condom Coloring Book" packed with 3D effect designs drawn by the inimitable prophylactic doodler Johnnie Jazzemup. Use you own creative talents to spice up these 55 assorted drawings with scintillating colors of your very own choosing.

# Credits

Thanks to Johnnie Jazzemup who came up this book idea. Thanks as well to Connie Doms for all your fantastic condom cartoons, most of them with their tongues hanging out, and thanks and condolences to Ivor Phewlines for all your futile attempts to garner literary recognition in this and other books that shall remain nameless and unsold.

And of course, let's not forget to thank our bird and bee friends, for without their tireless dedication to their momentous and fulfilling mission this book might not have been necessary.

> Bye for now folks...
> Thanks for visiting, Please come again whenever you feel up for it !

**The Cool Condom Compendium**

Copyright © 2018 Published by Jazzemup Creations

All rights reserved. No part of this book may be reproduced or transmitted in any form or by any means without written permission from the author.

ISBN-13: 978-0-9906975-5-8

Printed in USA by Create Space

www.ingramcontent.com/pod-product-compliance
Lightning Source LLC
Chambersburg PA
CBHW081017040426
42444CB00014B/3239